Foreword

People typically come to yoga looking for something they can't quite describe. Maybe it's strength, both physical and mental; maybe it's flexibility—again, both physical and mental. Maybe it's something to nourish their spirit and make them feel calmer and more capable of handling whatever comes their way.

The 4S Method takes that yoga wisdom and runs with it; it gives you strength drills for real life, suppleness for stiff mornings, and serenity hacks for chaotic days. It's like yoga's rebellious cousin who refuses to choose between one or the other. What you'll learn in this book is the 4S approach to folding *all* of these important elements into your life. It includes and moves beyond yoga, but it shares the same goal, moving you toward balance, freedom, and connection.

As you'll read, Holly first came to me to study how to teach yoga to athletes. Many students in that program initially think, "Athletes need to win! Let's make yoga tough to harden them up!" But they need exactly the opposite. Yoga for athletes is not athletic yoga.

Many in the general population come to yoga to build comfort with discomfort, to push their edges. But athletes are already trained to do that at the highest level. What athletes need is to build comfort with comfort: to be OK with just being OK, with staying far back from the fiery edge.

After many years of pushing her body toward its limits and paying the price for her zeal, Holly realized that's what she needed, too. And shifting her perspective on rest and recovery has helped turn her into an accidental wellness rebel. (Turns out, aging well isn't about grinding harder; it's about rewiring everything we've been taught.)

Holly generously shares her compelling personal story here. You'll likely recognize yourself in her journey: encountering a frustrating constellation of symptoms, only to be passed from practitioner to practitioner and being told "this is par for the course" for working moms.

But, like Holly, you know that's not true. You know there's something more for you. You know you can feel strong, supple, sustained, and serene. Holly will give you the tools to get there.

And when you do, you'll have:

1. *Strength.* We have to be strong as mothers—as *people* living in the world these days. You'll discover easy ways to keep yourself strong so you can show up fully for yourself and the people in your life. Her Pocket Movements reveal the radical truth: Wellness doesn't require hours of your time. These micro-practices contain all the essential elements—strength, mobility, recovery, and regulation—distilled into moments that actually fit real life.

2. *Suppleness*. By paying attention to your body's mobility and flexibility, you'll also develop your mental and emotional resilience and equanimity. Tuning in to your body gives you a pathway right to your soul.
3. *Sustenance*. Adopt a simple approach to nourishing yourself that reduces inflammation and sets you up for a long and comfortable life.
4. *Serenity*. By finding the right balance between work and rest, between effort and ease, you'll be better equipped to come back to a calm center, no matter what's going on in your life.

Best of all, when you follow the path Holly sets out here, you'll be more nourished and balanced, and thus far better able to do the work of supporting those around you, from aging parents and growing children to communities that need you.

Holly is a warm, kind, and present guide both in person and in writing. You're in great hands with her wide array of skills and life experience. She has walked the walk and is here to talk you toward this sweet spot of balance. She meets you where you are with her Pocket Movements, giving you tools to improve on every level. Holly knows a little can go a long way—and you will, too!

Be well!
Sage Rountree, PhD, E-RYT500

Praise for The Good Living Code

"The Good Living Code is a concise guide with practical wisdom for anyone seeking a healthier, more mindful, and more energized life. Holly's approach is approachable, actionable, and rooted in years of experience teaching movement and wellness."

- Tiffany Cruikshank, L.Ac, MAOM, founder of Yoga Medicine®

"Bringing together science, spirituality, and fitness, Holly Bonvissuto's The Good Living Code is an excellent roadmap for living well in an aging body."

- Sharon Salzberg, author of Lovingkindness and Real Change

Holly's 4S Method is a doable, repeatable, and enjoyable program that will make a transformational shift in your life. Changes will happen physically, emotionally and energetically with consistent application of the fundamental truths in this book. Combining scientifically backed principles with Holly's real-world experience you will move forward in becoming stronger and more resilient while having fun along the way.
I highly recommend The Good Living Code to help you live your best life.

- Dr. Perry Nickelston, DC, founder Stop Chasing Pain

"Holly Bonvissuto brings together decades of personal experience, as a mother, teacher, coach, and lifelong mover, with science-backed principles and a deeply compassionate approach. Rather than offering quick fixes, she lays out a sustainable framework built on four essential pillars: strength, suppleness, sustenance, and serenity. Her guidance is practical, grounding, and genuinely doable, even amid real-life chaos. The Pocket Movements Library is a standout feature: simple, bite-sized practices designed for busy days and low-energy moments. This book doesn't just teach you how to take care of yourself for the next month; it shows you how to build a way of living that supports you for decades to come."

- Dr. Diane Malaspina, M.S.Ed., PhD

Introduction

About 30 years ago, when I first met my husband, I learned his last name—Bonvissuto—which, loosely translated, means "well-lived" or "good living," from the Italian *buono* for good and *vissuto* for lived. At the time, it felt like a beautiful coincidence, but over the years, it's come to feel more like a calling.

When I took on this name, it wasn't just a change on paper; it became a quiet promise to myself. A vow to not just move through life, but to live it *well*. To weather its inevitable storms with grace, to find healing through hardship and to seek out joy, connection, and meaning even in the mundane.

That quiet promise eventually became the foundation of my business, Good Living Wellness. I chose that name not because I've mastered the art of "good living," but because I believe it's a journey we're all on. A lifelong practice of listening inward, honoring the wisdom of our bodies, tending to our energy, and choosing, again and again, to live with intention.

To me, "good living" isn't about chasing perfection. It's about presence. It's about reclaiming our vitality and worth, even in a world that often pulls us away from both. And it's about walking that path together with curiosity, compassion, and a commitment to live as fully and as well as we can.

This book is my love letter to that pursuit. To the small, daily choices that compound into a life of strength, suppleness, nourishment, and peace. To showing up—not for the perfect version of wellness, but for the version that lets us feel fully alive, exactly as we are.

There were too many years where I chased wellness like it was a finish line, pushing through fatigue, ignoring pain, and treating my body like a machine that should perform on demand. Then life forced me to stop. These were my lessons; they became my harsh teachers. I learned that real health isn't about brute force or quick fixes. It's about listening to the whispers (or shouts) of your body and responding with four essential gifts: *strength* to protect, *suppleness* to adapt, *sustenance* to nourish, and *serenity* to heal. Together, they form what I call the 4S Method, a framework forged from the crucible of my own brokenness and built through science, sustainability, and self-compassion.

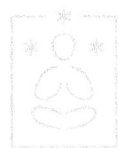

The Good Living Code is the book I needed when I was sick, scared, and lacking balance. It's about creating a life in which wellness, sustained through realistic habits, seeps into the cracks of your real, messy days and into the pockets of your time.

In these pages, I share with you the 4S Method, a foundational reset for approaching wellness that is both rewarding and sustainable. No surprise, it's not a quick fix. With it, you won't be chasing isolated metrics like steps, calories, and scale numbers, adopting some crazy wellness fad, or getting stuck in the damaging mindset that thinks fitness is "all-or-nothing."

With the 4S method, you learn to engage all the pieces that truly matter. You build a body that moves with ease, nourish yourself in ways that sustain energy, and cultivate a nervous system that's resilient enough to handle life's ups and downs and twists and turns. Whether you're navigating midlife transitions, postpartum recovery, empty nesting, or the surprises of aging, the 4S method creates a foundation designed to meet your ever-changing needs.

While I'm not a doctor—and this isn't medical advice—*The Good Living Code* blends peer-reviewed science, my professional training in yoga, mobility coaching, holistic wellness, and thousands of hours guiding clients through intelligent and sustainable movement and wellness practices. It's also rooted in my own journey through health challenges, parenting demands, and the hard-won realization that true wellness meets you exactly where you are.

This book is for people who don't want to just "snap back"; they want to *move forward* in life—gracefully, steadily, and with the feeling of strength and peace that lasts. If that's you, whether you're in your 40s, 50s, 60s or beyond, I want you to know that it's not too late to feel good in your body and your life.

This is wellness that doesn't demand that you stay forever young. This equips you to thrive and feel alive in every chapter of your life, exactly as you are.

 As you read, you'll learn to understand the importance of cultivating strength in your body, steadiness in your mind, and that profound sense of being at home in yourself—no matter your age or when you begin. This is what wellness truly means: good living as a daily practice, not a destination. It's moving through life with resilience, finding joy in capability, and resting in the deep self-trust that comes from listening to your body's wisdom.

A Moment to Arrive: Opening Practice

Settle into your body now. Close your eyes or soften your gaze.
Breathe in deeply... exhale slowly. Again. Breath in, breath out.

Notice here.
No need to fix. No need to rush.
You are here. You are enough.

Scan gently from your head to your toes.
Meeting tension with kindness,
Strength with gratitude.

Whisper silently:
"I am where I need to be.
I begin again. Now."

When you're ready, open your eyes.
Feel the ground. Feel your breath.
Welcome.

To support your practice, I've created exclusive companion audio for the meditations in this book. Scan the QR code or visit:
https://goodliving-wellness.com/my-book

Chapter 1
IT'S NOT TOO LATE

Sometimes the bravest and most important thing you can do is just show up.
— Brené Brown

You might be reading this because something has shifted in you. Because you hit a certain number of years. Because a stiffness lingered too long. Or because you had a moment in front of the mirror that made you ask, "How did I get *here*?"

Maybe your energy is unpredictable. Maybe your workouts don't function the way they used to. Maybe you've tried a few trending wellness offerings that promised transformation, only to find yourself exhausted, overwhelmed, or just... over it. Maybe you've discovered your "quick floor sit" to play with the dog now requires a strategic exit plan.

But you're not looking to become someone new, you're longing to feel like yourself again. Maybe, for the first time, you're wanting to truly feel at home in your body.

However you got here, I see you. Because I've lived these moments, too—in many different iterations.

I created the 4S Method to help people like you. People who are ready to take care of themselves—not just to *look* better, but to *live* better. And not just for the next 30 days, but for the next 30+ *years*.

These aren't theories. This method is built from my lived experience as a mother, teacher, coach, wellness seeker, and woman in motion through decades of change. It's infused with science-backed principles, practical tools, and most importantly, compassion. I've taught this method in yoga studios, corporate spaces, community forests, and one-on-one sessions—and now, I'm bringing it to you.

I'll walk you, step by step, through the four foundational principles of the 4S Method—what I call the four "pillars"—*strength*, *suppleness*, *sustenance*, and *serenity*. I'll also introduce you to my Pocket Movements Library—bite-sized movement practices I created for real life. Perfect for when your schedule is packed, your energy is low, or you just need something effective without overthinking it. These short sessions help you move with intention, even on the busiest or most unpredictable days.

While 45-minute classes and intense workout plans may have their place, I know from experience that what most people need is an easy, accessible way to get started or restarted, even when time is short and motivation is low. And a way to keep showing up, no matter your age, schedule, or story. A way that fits even when you are striving for the minimum and not the maximum on any given day. A way that sees how hard you push and offers you balance—not burnout.

This is your invitation to redefine what it means to age well. Not according to unrealistic ideals or aggressive routines, but by listening, honoring, and responding to your body with curiosity and care.

You don't need to overhaul your life. You don't need to chase youth. You need a rhythm that supports where you are now and all the moments that lie ahead. One that builds a foundation for durability, resilience, and freedom of movement. One that nourishes you deeply and creates more space for peace and ease to settle within you. This isn't about anti-aging—because time cannot be defeated. It's about *good living*.

Chapter 2
MY WORK CHOSE ME

The wound is the place where the light enters you.
– Rumi

I was a teacher, a runner, and a mom who did everything "right." I followed the rules, checked the boxes, and kept all my plates spinning.

Until one day, my body refused to play along.

In 2011, I travelled with my husband and our two boys to Mexico for my stepdaughter's wedding. I was looking forward to the time off, but instead of feeling full of sunshine and celebration, I was coughing a lot, and I felt feverish and thoroughly drained. Once I got back home, I felt like I had been hit by a Mack truck, and I was soon diagnosed with a double ear infection, impacted sinuses, and upper *and* lower respiratory infections. Still, my default is to press on and push through, so I kept going. Teaching. Running. Parenting. Nonstop. The antibiotics piled up, but the symptoms never really cleared. And I never truly got better.

One day, about a handful of months later, I came home from a long run and discovered a rash. I assumed it was from my shorts, so I didn't do anything about it. But within days, it grew into something far worse—an angry, blistering pain that wrapped around my hip and down my leg. It was shingles. And it was excruciating! It was worse than my Csections! I had to spend ten days at home wearing nothing but an oversized T-shirt; even fabric touching my skin was unbearable.

But an even bigger shock came shortly after my shingles outbreak, during a routine gynecological appointment. My doctor took one look at it, looked back at me, and said, "Holly, this is not normal for a 42-year-old."

Her words jolted me. I'd been telling myself for years that I was just worn down, just overextended, that everything I was feeling was temporary and fixable with more rest or willpower. But something in her tone cut through that denial. I opened up and shared with her more of my health history and experiences to date. She didn't pretend to have all the answers, but it was enough for her to pause, take me seriously, and run more tests than any doctor had before. When results were ready, my ANA test came back positive, which indicated my immune system was producing antibodies that were mistakenly attacking my own healthy cells—often a sign of autoimmune activity. But my OB-GYN didn't stop there. She contacted my primary care physician directly and urged him to dig deeper. That moment didn't solve everything, but it cracked something open in me—a sense that my concerns mattered and that my health was truly being taken seriously. For the first time, I felt seen and supported, and I finally began to trust myself, to advocate for my body, and to approach my wellness with a new sense of possibility.

A few days later, there was more news, and it was worse. My PCP left me an urgent voicemail at the school where I was teaching: "Call our office back as soon as possible," he insisted. Waiting until class was over so I could get to the front office was excruciating. When I finally called from the school secretary's office, he didn't mince words.

"Your tests indicate you might have cancer, Holly. We need to run more diagnostics."

The office around me blurred. My heart raced. I thought of my husband, our two little boys, and the possibility that I might not be around to raise them. It felt like a seismic shift within me. I knew in my bones that something had to change and that I couldn't ignore what my body had been trying to tell me: Something was very wrong.

The next few months became a blur of tests, referrals, and anxiety. Cancer was ruled out, but then came the suspicion of multiple sclerosis. Another dead end. A neurologist listened politely to my symptoms, looked me in the eyes, and told me, "You're a working mom. This is just par for the course." He handed me a prescription for antidepressants and muscle relaxers.

I was stunned. Then furious. After everything I'd been through—the months of unrelenting symptoms, the dead ends, the subtle and not-so-subtle gaslighting—and this was their answer? A pat on the head and a dismissal? For a split second, I almost turned on myself. Maybe I *was* being dramatic. Maybe this *was* just stress.

Then something deeper in me rose up—a kind of primal defiance. I wasn't broken, I realized. The system was. And if the system wasn't going to see me, I'd stop trying to be seen by it. So I stopped chasing validation from doctors who weren't listening, who weren't understanding, and I started forging my own path toward healing. It wasn't a polished plan, but it was a line in the sand. I wasn't going to be dismissed again. I knew in my heart there was a way to feel "normal" and, come hell or high water, I would find it.

I reached out to a trusted friend and naturopath and began to dig deeper. Together, we discovered and addressed inflammation as well as an overgrowth of systemic Candida, a fungal overgrowth in the body that can disrupt digestion, hormones, immunity, and energy levels. She also introduced me to a few ways to support my immune system to help it fight back.

I became obsessed with learning. I read, researched, and eventually enrolled in a program to become a board-certified holistic health coach. The work gave me several things I had been missing, and I learned a few important tools. And I began to learn to trust myself. I was receiving a deeper understanding, a way to participate in my healing.

Through that journey, I gained a new relationship with my body, one rooted in curiosity instead of frustration. I began to understand not just the *what* of my symptoms but the *why* behind them. I learned how stress, sleep, movement, food, and thoughts were all woven together in the landscape of health. My body stopped feeling like something I had to push and became something I could support. I discovered how to listen more deeply, to notice subtle signals before they became loud symptoms. I learned how to nourish my body in ways that felt sustainable, not punishing. That shift gave me agency. It gave me choices. It gave me the tools to stop outsourcing my well-being and start working in partnership with myself.

In 2024, after exhaustion, joint pain, and some brain fog flared up yet again, and followed by another round of bloodwork, I finally received a real diagnosis. It was lupus. In an unexpected way, it brought me relief. A name gave me something to work with. And thanks to the path I'd already been walking, I had the tools I needed.

All of the lessons I had learned up to that point, through formal training and lived experience, came into focus. I knew how to read my body's signals and respond early. I knew how to reduce inflammation through nutrition, regulate my nervous system through breath and movement, and support detoxification through hydration, lymphatic flow, and rest. I understood how to pull back when needed, without guilt, and how to best support myself instead of pushing through. These weren't abstract wellness concepts; they were the very practices that helped prevent this flare up from spiraling out of control.

Even in the absence of immediate solutions from doctors, I wasn't helpless. I wasn't starting from zero. I knew how to stabilize my system and how to create an internal environment where healing could begin. It wasn't necessarily easy, but I had a direction to move toward—and the ability to influence my own outcome.

This reminded me that an important part of the work of being well isn't about perfection. It's about *resilience*. When life knocks you for a loop—and it will—you need a foundation strong enough to help you return to center. Resilience is necessary to keep showing up for yourself, especially in the messy, uncomfortable moments. It's what allows you to keep choosing healing, even when things feel hard or progress feels slow. It's the quiet commitment to keep tending to your body, mind, and spirit—not just when things are going well, but through the highs and lows, the flare-ups and setbacks.

After all, wellness isn't a final destination. It's the repeated daily practice of remembering you have a choice, and choosing to care for yourself again and again.

Enter Yoga

My introduction to yoga—and the healing journey it launched—didn't start with something as lofty as ambition or motivation. No, I started yoga because my OB-GYN at the time suggested it would help me connect better with my body. I'd had four miscarriages, and I needed to try something different. So, in 2000, I stepped into a prenatal yoga class, and, to my surprise, it was the gateway to an entirely new perspective and would later shape my entire approach to wellness.

At the time, I wasn't looking for spiritual awakening or transformation. I just wanted to feel something, anything, other than disconnection and defeat! That first class awakened me to more than the ability to move again. It gave me presence. It gave me permission to slow down. And it gave me a new kind of relationship with my body, one that wasn't purely medical or mechanical—but mindful.

After all, for so long, my body and mind had been in a constant battle, one I didn't even realize I was fighting. I was tense, guarded, always bracing for the next loss or disappointment. My nervous system had forgotten how to feel safe. Through yoga, though, I began to experience small moments of relief, where breath and movement created just enough space for a truce. Over time, it felt like my body and mind were learning to speak the same language again—not as enemies, but as allies. They were finally on the same side. Mine.

Yoga began to teach me that movement could be medicine. It taught me that the breath could be a bridge between chaos and calm. And later, as I wound my way through illness, motherhood, grief, and the long journey home to myself, an even deeper learning blossomed within me. Yoga taught me how to inhabit my body with compassion. Instead of seeing my body as something broken or burdensome, I began to witness it as something worthy of care, something wise, resilient, and responsive. That inner shift didn't just guide my healing; it changed the way I showed up for myself and others. It opened a door to the path I walk today.

Today, I work with people navigating their own storms—parents, caregivers, professionals. People who feel the weight of responsibilities and the frustration of their bodies not feeling like their own. And I understand them deeply because I've been there. Like them, I've endured "normal" lab tests alongside persistent fatigue. Like them, I've pushed my body toward perfection, only to succumb to it pushing back as it refused to take any more. Like many of them, I've looked fine on the outside while barely holding it together on the inside.

That's why my expertise isn't only professional, it's personal. It's lived. I've walked through the confusion, the setbacks, the fear of not knowing what's wrong or how to fix it. And because of that, I'm able to meet others with empathy, not just protocols. This work didn't just call to me; I lived my way into it. It found me in the middle of my own healing, and now I get to walk alongside others as they find their way back to wellness. And that lights me up. I get to help people move better, feel stronger, age vibrantly, and be empowered to build a sustainable foundation that supports their well-being year after year after year.

Here's my invitation to you:

Get curious about your well-being
Believe in the possibility of healing
Stop chalking everything up to aging
Remember: Your body isn't the enemy
Your body is the messenger
It is time to start listening

Reflection:
When have you felt dismissed by a doctor or loved one? How did it shape your self-advocacy?

Chapter 3
YOGA TO HIIT AND BACK AGAIN

You can't outperform your nervous system.
– Dr. Kelly Starrett

After I completed my holistic health coaching certification, I dove into learning everything I could about natural health—how to support the body's healing through nutrition, movement, stress management, plant-based remedies, and other alternative approaches that nurture balance and vitality. I paused my running routine so I could focus on healing, and I fully committed myself to yoga. I practiced as many days a week as I could.

Around that time, my family and I made the decision to downsize and move to a different part of the Atlanta suburbs, one that would be closer to my husband's work. The move would also grant me the opportunity to focus more on my health—and I wouldn't need to teach. The downside, however, was that I didn't yet have a community or any close friends in the area. (Just for reference, if you move 30 minutes from friends with kids in Atlanta, you might as well be in a different state. "Long-distance" local relationships cannot survive the Atlanta traffic!)

So, after living in a supportive neighborhood, enjoying deep friendships for 13 years, the contrast wasn't just jarring; it was heartbreaking. I felt untethered. It was a lonely, disorienting time. I was being strong for my husband and our sons, and I put on a brave face, but I felt bereft. It was a lonely time for me. My kids were in fourth and seventh grade, ages that meant there weren't as many easy opportunities for me to connect with other parents as there'd been when my kids were in preschool. I hadn't expected the move to feel like such a rupture, but it did. I missed my people. I missed being known. I didn't realize how much of a loss I would feel, and I soon longed for community. I tried a few gyms and yoga studios, but I struggled in my new environment.

Strength Alone Isn't Enough

By January 2018, I was feeling stronger and healthier, and I joined a local women's boot camp. I loved the structured workouts, the sense of challenge, and the camaraderie, which brought me some much-needed connection. I began to make a few dear friends and felt like I was finally finding my footing. But I didn't realize the toll that six days a week of HIIT plus weight training was taking on my body. I was *strong*—but I was brittle.

I started to learn that *strength* without *suppleness* is like a sheet of glass: it's solid—until it cracks.

In the meantime, I was in perimenopause; I didn't yet understand the physiological shifts that were occurring beneath the surface. Fluctuating hormones can increase inflammation, reduce our capacity for recovery, and impair our sleep. No one had told me that high-intensity training without adequate rest can worsen those conditions and even lead to injury, burnout, and hormonal dysregulation. So, I kept pushing. I kept doing what I thought I should be doing, only with more effort, more sweat, and more intensity, believing that discipline—and the more of it, the better—would eventually lead to results. But instead of feeling stronger, I felt more depleted. My body was trying to get my attention, but I wasn't listening.

In addition to boot camp, I resumed my running, and yoga was gradually taking a back seat. I was already hardwired to push myself, but at boot camp, the message was clearly delivered: "Go harder." "Go all in." "No pain, no gain." I was overtraining and under-recovering, and I didn't have mobility practices or true rest days built into my schedule. I wasn't doing anything to support joint health, tissue resilience, or nervous system regulation; it was just grind and *go*.

I was intoxicated by the sense of belonging and achievement, but I didn't know what I didn't know. I didn't realize that training without recovery was actually breaking me down. I didn't yet understand how to train *smarter* instead of just *harder*.

Not surprisingly, the injuries came fast and furious. First, I strained my rotator cuff, then I strained my quadratus lumborum (QL). Then I struggled with tendonitis in my hip. Not too long after healing from that, I was on a trail run, and the ligaments in one very weakened ankle tore up.

With each setback, my body was surely asking me to pause and reassess, but I wasn't listening. Once my ankle fell apart, though, I had no choice *but* to listen. I couldn't bear any weight on my left side. I was forced to stop everything and take a pause.

My physical therapist was blunt with me, and I finally heard what I hadn't been letting in: "Holly, you have got to stop." I didn't want to hear it! But I relented. I took some time to heal and found my way back to the practice I had drifted from, the practice I had cherished: *yoga*. And when I finally stepped back onto the mat, I began to remember what I had loved so deeply about it. It wasn't just the movement. It wasn't just the poses. It was the *presence*, the *breath*, the *grounding*.

I found a local yoga studio and became a member. My kids were a bit older by then, and I finally felt I had the space to pursue something I had longed to do: enroll in a yoga teacher training course. I had looked into it at that first studio I'd gone to 19 years before, but life had felt too chaotic back when my boys were little. Spending 200 hours away from my small children felt like far too big of an ask—for my husband, for my boys, and for me, too. Now that they were older (one in college, the other in high school), it felt like the right time. I was ready to learn why being on my mat always made me feel welcome—like returning home—no matter how long I'd been away!

I loved everything about the 200-hour yoga teacher training course I enrolled in. I was especially grateful for the friendships I was cultivating. Immediately after finishing my 200 hours, I signed up for an intensive with Sage Rountree in her Yoga for Athletes training at Kripalu Center for Yoga & Health in Stockbridge, Massachusetts. I had read some of her books a while back and appreciated her practical, compassionate approach to yoga.

Sage's training inspired another lightbulb moment. It dawned on me what had been missing from the boot camp world I'd been immersed in—I didn't yet have a way to build in active recovery to my workouts. Active recovery is a gentle, intentional way to help your body recover after working out by moving it *just enough*. Instead of complete rest, like spending the day on the couch, it involves low-intensity movement that restores rather than depletes.

When we move gently, we keep blood and lymph flowing, which brings nutrients to our muscles and helps flush out waste. This kind of movement supports circulation, reduces soreness and stiffness, promotes faster healing, and helps us return to a state of overall vitality and balance.

 I began to recognize that my body didn't need more *pushing*; it needed a smarter way to *recover*. It needed me to find a way to encourage performance without constantly pushing myself to the point of breaking. It needed *balance*. "Training tears you down; recovery builds you up," Sage writes in her book *The Athlete's Guide to Recovery*. Those words continue to inspire me.

So I kept an open mind and continued learning. I was incredibly curious about the practice I love, as well as these incredible human bodies we move around in. I dove into several advanced trainings. I took Myofascial Release Training, got trained as a Yoga Corrective Exercise Specialist, and worked to receive a 300-hour yoga teacher training certification. I trained in Restorative Yoga and Yoga Nidra. Each layer of learning deepened my understanding, not just of anatomy and alignment, but of how the nervous system, the mind, and the body interact as a whole. These practices weren't just physical; they were medicinal. I knew it. I felt it. I lived it.

This shift from pushing my body to partnering with it—weaving in more restorative practices to bring balance, sustainability, and deeper healing into my movement and my life—was profound. The more time I spent creating this balance, the clearer its importance became.

In 2024, I completed Level 1 and 2 of Mobility Training with Dr. Kelly Starrett, a physical therapist, movement expert, and author of *Becoming a Supple Leopard*, and it brought me another massive "a-ha" moment. All the pieces—all of my training—were clicking together like pieces of a puzzle. I loved the scientific approach of Kelly's mobility training, its clear strategies, and its focus on improving the *quality* of movement. "Your body is a systems-based machine," Kelly wrote in *Becoming a Supple Leopard*, "and all systems are interconnected."

I also read *Built to Move*, which Kelly wrote with his wife, Juliet, and I was impressed by their emphasis on foundational daily movement habits that support long-term mobility. They pointed out simple acts, like sitting on the floor, walking more, and reclaiming positions our bodies are meant to take naturally. These habits aren't extreme at all. In fact, they are essential to creating suppleness—when a body is both strong and mobile and is capable of moving freely, adapting to stress, and recovering with ease.

All Four Pieces in Place

As I trained with Kelly, I noticed another gap: most of the people he worked with were elite athletes, heavy weightlifters, or CrossFitters. But those aren't the people I usually serve. So, with Kelly's encouragement, I spent months thinking about how I might adapt his and other tools to be accessible to everyday people. People who, like me, tend to go all in on something and need a more balanced approach. People who are navigating real-life demands, dealing with hormonal changes, or managing chronic stress, injuries, or fatigue, but who are still ready and willing and even hungry to move with ease, feel strong, and age vibrantly.

Then it became my mission. I passionately wanted to bridge the gap between high-performance mobility strategies and accessible approaches to wellness. I wanted to create programming that focuses on strength and movement on the one hand, while, on the other hand, cultivates restoration and helps regulate the nervous system. I envisioned how combining yoga and breathwork with strength and mobility development could elevate all four of the practices. I wanted to offer something more than just a workout; I wanted to make available an intelligent, sustainable movement *system* that fosters longevity.

By that time, I had earned several different certifications and completed many trainings—health and wellness coaching, yoga, myofascial release, mobility training, personal training, mat and reformer Pilates—but my own body was still sending signals that something wasn't right. Between 2020 and 2025, life threw everything at me: a parathyroid tumor, my son's mental health crisis, the upheaval of menopause, and recurring autoimmune flare-ups. It was a storm that no single practice could weather alone. But something emerged from that period that wasn't just survival—it was a deeper integration of everything I'd studied. I began to weave together the essentials of strength, suppleness, sustenance, and serenity—not just for my clients, but for myself, too. And the 4S Method was born—not as a quick fix, but as a sustainable framework that helped me reclaim stability and vitality, even in the most demanding seasons of life.

By 2025, I had been teaching clients and leading workshops about how to age well, using all the pillars of what would become the 4S Method. I just hadn't thought to tie them together with a bow—until now. Aging well doesn't mean being free from struggle. It means building resilience, staying curious, and adapting with self-compassion. The 4S

Method wasn't born from perfection—it was born from necessity. I taught what I was actively practicing: using strength to stay steady, supporting suppleness to stay mobile, feeding sustenance to fuel recovery, and deepening serenity to find peace amidst it all.

The 4S Method is not a rigid protocol; it is an adaptive lens for holistic well-being. To age well, we must work all four of these principles. They are non-negotiable. At the same time, The 4S Method isn't a simple course in "wellness" as you've known it. It's a sustainable, interconnected system—one that honors how your body *actually* changes through seasons of stress, healing, and aging. And here's the best part: No matter where you are when you start, the 4S Method meets you there.

Ready to begin?

Reflection:
What's your version of overtraining? Where could balance feel like rebellion?

Chapter 4
THE 4S METHOD

"We do not rise to the level of our goals. We fall to the level of our systems."
— *James Clear*

Let's take a closer look at the four pillars of the 4S method. Remember each pillar matters, but it's their synergy that makes the 4S Method so effective.

Strength is your body's resilient response to life's demands. In the 4S Method, we cultivate durable power through joint-protective resistance training, yoga-inspired load-bearing postures, and recovery-focused progression. Strength isn't about aesthetics; it's about "functional vitality"—the ability to move and live with energy, ease, and resilience in everyday life. It protects our joints, supports bone health, and builds the resilience we need to hike, carry groceries, play with grandchildren, or simply move through daily life with confidence and ease. It's what allows us to keep doing the things that bring us joy, well into the future.

Suppleness is often mistaken for flexibility alone, but it's so much more. It refers to how well our bodies move and respond under load and across time. Suppleness is essential for aging with grace and agility. In the 4S Method, we develop suppleness through mobility practices, dynamic stretching, strength, and myofascial massage. When tissues are well-hydrated and mobile, we move more freely, adapt more quickly, and protect ourselves from injury. Suppleness helps us bend without breaking, both physically and metaphorically.

Sustenance forms the energetic foundation of vibrant aging. It's not just about what we eat, but how we nourish our bodies at the cellular level. In the 4S Method, sustenance focuses on anti-inflammatory foods, hydration that supports tissue health, and habits that restore metabolic efficiency. It's about fueling the body to reduce inflammation, support energy production, and give our systems what they need to heal, move, and thrive. True nourishment goes beyond food; it's an act of ongoing care and intention.

Serenity is the anchor of the entire method. Without a regulated nervous system, the other elements struggle to stick. Serenity gives the body permission to repair, recharge, and integrate. In the 4S Method, we cultivate serenity through breathwork, sleep, rest, meditation, stillness, and restorative movement. These practices strengthen emotional resilience and provide a sense of grounding, especially when life feels uncertain. Rest isn't something we earn after the hard work; it is the work. It's fundamental to healing, wholeness, and long-term well-being.

This isn't wellness as you've known it. It's a sustainable, interconnected system—one that honors how your body *actually* changes through seasons of stress, healing, and aging. And here's the best part: No matter where you are when you start, the 4S Method meets you there.

Systems Matter More Than Willpower

I used to believe that the most important factor in my own healing was discipline. I thought I needed to wake up at 5:30 a.m. for a good workout or some running, do a lot of meal prep, stick to an extreme calorie deficit or fast, and then feverishly grind away until I collapsed.

James Clear is known for his work on habit formation and behavior change. In his book *Atomic Habits,* he writes: "True behavior change is *identity* change. You might start a habit because of motivation, but the only reason you'll stick with one is that it becomes part of your identity."

The 4S Method is a holistic framework for vibrant aging, inspired from my journey through life and misdiagnosis, injury, chronic stress, menopause, and lupus. It isn't about willpower; it's about designing a life in which healthy choices feel inevitable. Willpower is like a muscle—and it can easily be too tired to lift one dumbbell or resist the siren call of a nearby couch. It's not anything we can rely on for our health over the long-term. That's why it's essential to have a system in place to build lasting change.

As I faced some undeniable truths in my own life, the 4S Method began to take shape. These truths hit hard:

- **The body speaks in patterns, not single symptoms.** I finally learned that my miscarriages, gut issues, migraines, and joint pain were all connected.
- **Life (especially midlife) requires flexibility, not rigidity.**

What worked when we're 30 or 40 often backfires at 45 or 55 due to hormonal shifts.
- **Simplicity leads to sustainability**.
  Small, consistent habits win every time.
- **Balance is not found in a static state.**
  Balance is the result of fluidity and adaptability. Because you do not achieve balance once, it is a perennial effort that is required through all life's changes.

The Science Behind the Synergy

Research shows that interconnected systems work best. A 2023 meta-analysis in *Maturitas* suggests that, for midlife women, multicomponent interventions—such as combining movement, nutrition, and stress management—can bring two to three times greater improvements over isolated approaches in outcomes, such as metabolic health and cognitive function.[1]

Dr. Lisa Mosconi is a leading neuroscientist and women's brain health specialist who directs the Women's Brain Initiative at Weill Cornell Medicine. Her research demonstrates that optimal health is achieved by physical activity, micronutrient-rich diets, such as Mediterranean-style eating, neural adaptability (supported by techniques like yoga Nidra), and stress resilience (via vagus nerve activation). These factors collectively modulate estrogen's neuroprotective effects.[2] Other studies show that dynamic mobility lubricates joints two times better than static holds.

At the same time, chronic stress, in fact, can physically shrink muscle cells.[3]

What's most important to notice is that the best results come from addressing multiple areas at once. Mosconi explains that hormonal health during midlife depends on four key factors:

- Regular movement (both aerobic and strength training)
- Micronutrient-rich foods (like Mediterranean diet staples)
- Brain flexibility (boosted by practices like yoga nidra)
- Stress resilience (through vagus nerve stimulation)

These elements work together to support estrogen's natural protective effects on the brain and body. Your body's systems are deeply connected; what helps your heart helps your brain, and stress management makes your workouts more effective.

The Synergy of the Four Pillars of Wellness

Unlike siloed approaches to wellness, the 4S Method integrates four pillars of wellness:

Strength—combating age-related muscle loss and reducing falls

Suppleness—prioritizing dynamic mobility over static stretching and incorporating myofascial release for pain-free movement.

Sustenance— staying adequately hydrated and using anti-inflammatory nutrition to heal the gut and reduce systemic inflammation

Serenity—regulating the nervous system through ensuring quality sleep and taking up practices like breathwork and yoga in one or more of its forms.

The 4S Method adapts to real-life challenges like hormonal shifts and time constraints. Instead of demanding hours of you that you don't have, it integrates into those stolen moments in your life—the time while your coffee brews, during TV ads, or in between meetings. It rejects rigid "anti-aging" rules in favor of sustainable micro-habits. It emphasizes setting up easy habits over a balls-to-the-wall mentality and favors monitoring body wisdom more than external metrics. Rooted in both clinical evidence and my lived experience, the 4S Method honors that strength, nourishment, mobility, and resilience intertwine to rewrite what's possible as we age.

The 4S Method is intended to help you design a life where healthy choices feel natural, not forced. Instead of fighting against your schedule or energy levels, you'll learn to tweak your surroundings so strength, nourishment, mobility, and resilience fit seamlessly into your day. As James Clear puts it: "You don't have to be the victim of your environment. You can also be the architect of it." Consider the 4S Method to be your toolkit for becoming that architect, on your terms, in your real life.

Reflection:
Which of the four pillars feels most nourished in your life? Which feels most neglected?

Chapter 5
STRENGTH – RECLAIMING YOUR POWER

*"Strong women aren't simply born.
They are made by the storms they walk through."*
— *Unknown*

I'll never forget the time I was having a lupus flare-up while I was making lunch in my kitchen. My hands were aching to the bone, and I was so terribly fatigued that I had to ask my son to open the lid of a jar for me. The woman who once easily powered through boot camp workouts six days a week was now struggling with something as simple as opening a pickle jar! In that vulnerability, I understood what real, lifelong strength meant. It wasn't just about powering through; it was about building a resilient foundation—one that offers stability and durability even on the hardest days. This is the strength that carries us forward. And that is the essence of the Strength pillar: learning to build resilience in a way that truly sustains you.

The Science Behind Strength Training Plus Yoga

As a yoga teacher, I see dedicated yogis every week who fold effortlessly into forward bends but then wobble uncontrollably in Warrior III. I also see students who flow gracefully through vinyasas yet struggle to rise from the floor without using their hands.

The flexibility and balance that yoga offers are very valuable, of course, but they don't offer the progressive resistance needed to combat age-related muscle loss.[4] A 2023 review of multiple studies found that yoga can help improve balance and leg strength in older adults, but pairing it with strength training, such as weight lifting, often leads to even greater benefits.[5]

Strength Protects Joints

When we sink into deep hip external rotation poses like Pigeon without enough hip mobility or glute engagement, the knee often ends up taking on extra strain. Over time, that added stress can increase injury risk. This connection is seen in both yoga injury research and studies on how lower-body alignment affects our joints. Strengthening your hip muscles, especially with exercises like banded clamshell workouts, can help build up your gluteus medius.[6, 7] Research shows that a stronger glute medius may ease lower back and hip pain, which is why these exercises are commonly used in rehab.[8]

Functional Strength = Real-Life Mobility

Lower-body resistance exercises significantly boost chair-stand performance, a key indicator of functional longevity.[9]

Better Balance

Studies show that adding exercises like heel raises and single-leg stands reduced fall risk by approximately 24–37% compared to yoga alone.[10]

Kelly Starrett agrees with these principles. He suggests that focusing solely on mobility exercises without addressing underlying stability issues may not be effective and could potentially be counterproductive or even dangerous. By building a solid foundation of stability through strength, you empower your body to access and control its full range of motion. This leads to improved quality movement, reduced risk of injury, and enhanced performance—on the yoga mat or wherever you find yourself moving.

The vinyasa classes I teach now are not fast-paced, although some might say they are challenging. With Kelly's philosophy in mind, I often integrate micro-strength drills into every class, for example:

- Half-lowering planks—providing eccentric strength
- Floating heels—providing ankle stability
- Pulses in Crescent Lunge—offering endurance and power

Beyond burning more calories at rest, muscle acts as a crucial protector for joints and overall health.[11] We know muscles help us move, but they have hidden superpowers, too. Muscle is a metabolically active tissue, which means it helps break down substances in the body for energy.[12] When the body is at rest, each pound of muscle burns 6-10 calories.[13] Furthermore, muscle acts like armor for the joints. It helps absorb impact from daily movements, from walking to running and everything in between. Muscles are also joint stabilizers, preventing misalignment and lowering risk of injury.[14]

Arthritis Relief

Research shows that resistance training—like using weights, resistance bands, or even your own bodyweight—can significantly reduce arthritis symptoms.[15] In fact, meta-analyses—large studies that combine results from many trials—have shown that people experience about 40 to 70% improvement in both pain and daily function.[16] That means strength training isn't just safe for arthritis, it can be one of the most effective ways to feel and move better.

Strength = Independence

Higher grip strength correlates with lower mortality risk and reduced hospitalization rates.[17] (To measure such things, you can get a handgrip dynamometer online, or you can notice if you can't hold your groceries for long without fatiguing.) And chair-stand test scores predict future mobility and quality of life more accurately than routine blood panels.[18]

The Hormone Connection

Perimenopausal women can lose muscle at nearly twice the typical rate—about six to 10% per decade.[19] Yet resistance exercise preserves substantially more muscle than cardio alone.[20]

It took time for me to piece everything together because my journey wasn't linear.

As I've mentioned, in 2018, six days a week of HIIT and training runs, left me injured, inflamed, and my cortisol levels were off the rails. In 2020, my yoga practice rebuilt my mind-body connection, but left me losing strength. In 2023, Pilates training revealed the power of controlled resistance. Now, I am blending yoga, bodyweight exercises, mat work, resistance bands, and weights for sustainable strength.

As I look back, the injuries and illnesses that used to feel like setbacks have become my greatest teachers. Each time, I dug a little deeper, learned a little more, and gave myself more grace. As Maya Angelou said, "Do the best you can until you know better. Then when you know better, do better." Every time, I set out to do better—not just for myself, but for my students and clients to help them do better, too.

Strength Training for Real Lives

Let's dismantle some of the misconceptions many of us have bought into:
- **"I need heavy weights"**
  Bodyweight and resistance bands can build remarkable strength. Building to heavy weights is an option, with all the other components in place.
- **"I don't have time"**
  Two 15-minute sessions per week can produce significant benefits[21,22]

- **"I'm too injured"**
  Yoga and Pilates adaptations prove there's always a safe way forward.

Client Spotlight

I asked Holly to create for me the yoga routine that would address my multiple orthopedic problems and limitations, as well as to improve the muscle tone and reduce the level of pain. I had been very impressed by the outcome of her creative approach. The routine movements and tools she recommended gave me possibilities to easily apply them a few times a day. They are fun to do, and I feel much better than before.
Holly is such an emphatic, attentive, and knowledgeable teacher, giving her extensive yoga experience for the benefit of every person looking for a healthier and pain-free life.
D.M.

Good living isn't about getting "ripped"—it's about lifting your grandchildren. Carrying your groceries without pain. Opening up your own damn jars.

Strength matters—especially after 40. That's because, starting around 40, our bodies typically face:

- 3 to 5% decline in muscle mass (*sarcopenia*) per decade[23]
- Bone density loss—especially in women[24]
- Slowed metabolic efficiency[25]

Research shows that resistance training can counteract these declines.

- Lifting weights two to three times a week can increase your spine's bone density by approximately 2-3% over eight months.[26]
- Strength training reduces fall risk by around 28%.[27]
- "Exercise snacks" (e.g., calf raises) may help with blood sugar management.[28]
- Even individuals in their 90s can build strength via light resistance work.[29]
- Combined strength training and nutritional programs can reverse frailty.[30]

Here's what I recommend you include to get your practice going. They work for me and my clients!

- **Work with resistance bands**. They are portable, adaptable, and perfect for travel.
- **Include mat work**. As of late, mat work is where I find the most joy in strength work. And my clients report they feel empowered by it.
- **Practice Pocket Movements**. *Pocket Movements*™ are short (13 minutes or less) strength sessions, and they fit in the pockets of your time. For example, you can do calf raises while you're brushing your teeth. I talk about this in detail on Chapter 9.

Getting Started

Strength training doesn't require a gym or perfect conditions. Start where you are.

- **Bodyweight basics.** Squats, push-ups, lunges—against a wall or on your knees if needed—and seated leg lifts build foundational strength.

- **Resistance bands.** These are portable and adaptable for travel or small spaces. Try banded rows or glute bridges.
- **Functional Movements.** Train for daily life—practice sitting-to-standing from a chair (no hands!) or carrying groceries evenly.

Start your first week with micro-sessions. Take two 10-minute strength breaks weekly, such as doing calf raises while brushing your teeth or doing wall sits during phone calls.

Remember that no matter how many times you stop, it is never too late to start again. Research shows that strength training, even just twice a week, can rebuild fragile muscles and reverse frailty in older adults. One powerful study found that when seniors combined simple resistance exercises with proper nutrition for just 12 weeks, 63% reversed their frailty completely. That's nearly double the improvement seen in those who didn't follow the program![31]

Finally, focus on *controlled movements* rather than rushing through reps. For example, when sitting into a chair, lower yourself slowly (aim for three seconds down), pause briefly at the bottom, then push up steadily (about one second up). This builds strength safely and teaches your body proper movement patterns.

And remember to track your wins. What feels easier? Climbing stairs? Carrying a laundry basket? Progress is personal.

Reflection:
What daily task do you want to do effortlessly in 10 years? How can you train for it now?

Chapter 6
SUPPLENESS – MOVING WITH EASE

"If you don't find time to take care of your body, you'll be forced to make time for your illness."
— *Robin Sharma*

We aren't meant to shrink with age; we're meant to deepen. Suppleness gives us the capacity to bend without breaking, to stretch into new versions of ourselves, and to age with vitality.

Suppleness isn't just a nice thing to have, it's something we need to have for vibrant aging. That's why it's the second pillar of the 4S Method.

Suppleness creates a foundation for graceful aging. My husband and I—I'm 55, and he's a few steps ahead of me at 66—often talk about the kind of life we want to lead into our 70s, 80s, and beyond. We're not looking to simply *exist*; we want to thrive—to hike, travel, and move without pain or fear of injury. Suppleness, our body's ability to move with fluidity and resilience, is central to that goal.

In the 4S Method, suppleness has to do with our relationship with mobility, flexibility, and the health of our fascial system. While strength gives us power and structure, sustenance nourishes and hydrates us. Where serenity grounds us, suppleness plays behind the scenes to keep everything moving well. Without it, aging becomes stiff, brittle, and more prone to injury and burnout.

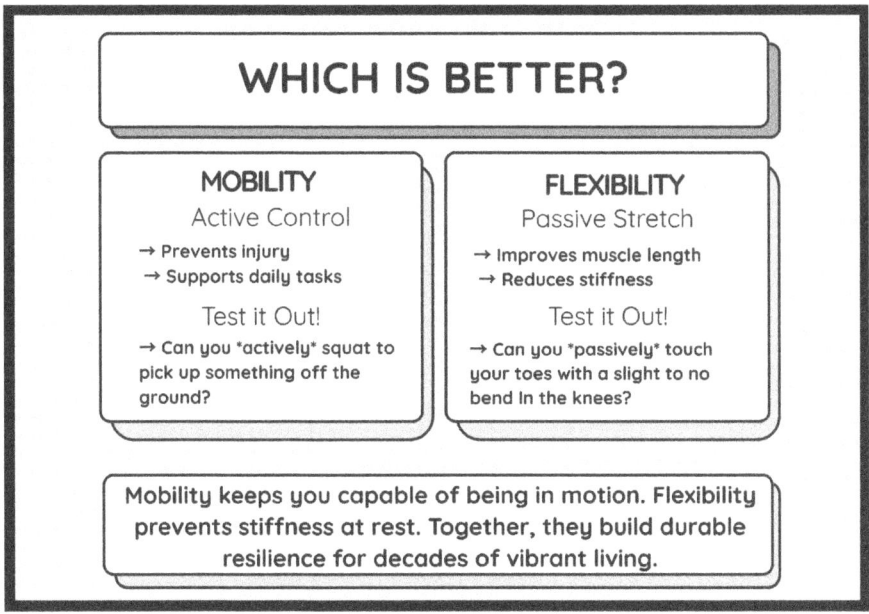

My Journey Through the Layers of Fascia and Flow

My interest in fascia began in earnest when I completed Jill Miller's Roll Model Method training in 2020, and it significantly changed how I understood the body. I had been teaching yoga for just a short while, and I knew regular myofascial release practices, such as rolling with therapy balls, would be a powerful agent for change. But this took it to a new level.

If you are not familiar with it, *fascia* is the stretchy, web-like tissue that wraps around and connects nearly all of your body's structures—muscles, bones, organs, and nerves—

keeping everything in place while allowing smooth movement. It's made of strong, flexible fibers that act like a body-wide support system, and it helps transmit a force that acts like shock absorbers when you exercise, walk, jump, or fall. Fascia is rich with nerve endings and carries sensory information that helps you sense things like pressure, tension, pain, and even where your body is in space. Sometimes, it even sends sensory signals, such as pain or stiffness.

When your fascia is healthy, it glides easily, but dehydration, lack of movement, or injury can make it sticky or tight, leading to pain and restricted motion. Caring for fascia through hydration, stretching, and movement keeps your body resilient, mobile, and pain-free.

After I added a twice-weekly rolling class to my teaching schedule, I noticed something extraordinary happening for students who attended regularly: they were transforming. In these students, long-held patterns of pain shifted and dissolved. Shoulders softened. Hips opened. Breath deepened. Students who had plateaued in their flexibility or carried chronic stiffness began to feel real change. And the magic? It wasn't from deeper stretching; it was from focused attention on the fascia.

Jill Miller writes in her book, *The Roll Model*: "Fascia is the seam system of your body, the missing link in modern movement and manual therapy." The science supported what I was seeing.

But it wasn't until I studied with Kelly Starrett and completed both levels of his Mobility Coach training in 2024 that I understood how to take these concepts even further. Kelly's work emphasizes a performance-based, accessible approach to mobility that empowers everyday people, not just athletes. "All human beings should be able to perform basic maintenance on themselves," Kelly wrote in *Becoming a Supple Leopard.*

His mentorship helped me synthesize the work I'd been doing with yoga and rolling into a system that focused not only on recovery but on performance and longevity. This clarity birthed a new offering: a special Flow + Mobility class that integrates yoga flow, functional movement, and dynamic mobility. It's become one of my most popular and beloved offerings. Students tell me they feel stronger *and* more mobile, more capable and more confident in their bodies.

Think of suppleness as a function of fascial health. Because the fascia —the body-wide connective tissue network — must be stimulated through regular movement to remain hydrated and glide freely, preventing the stiffness associated with aging; suppleness is a critical component to aging well. It is what maintains your functional independence—allowing you to move freely without pain—by ensuring your body's internal connective tissue remains resilient and adaptable, not stiff and restrictive.

Client Spotlight

"I have been doing Roll and Restore [myofascial massage with Restorative Yoga] with Holly for several years. When I started class, I had chronic back pain. In my daily life, I sit at a computer, which adds to my issues. For me, this practice has been immensely helpful in releasing muscle tension and reducing my back discomfort. I now have increased my mobility and range of motion. My overall physical health and mental calmness have improved. Holly's knowledge of the anatomy, holistic guidance, and care have taught me how to take better care of myself. I will follow all that she has taught me for the rest of my life.
S.W.

The Link Between Feelings, Fluidity, and Fascia

What I've come to believe deeply, and what the research supports, is that stiffness isn't just physical. Emotional experiences often embed themselves into our tissues, especially the fascia. Trauma, stress, and emotional holding can create literal knots in our mobility.

A 2022 study explored the association between fascia thickness and flexibility in older adults and found that thickened, dehydrated fascia is linked to decreased joint mobility and a higher risk of movement limitations as we age.[32]

The data reinforced something I've long sensed in my students: that lack of movement isn't just a symptom of aging—it's a *cause*. And it's *reversible*.

When I guide clients through a fascia-based practice, I often see more than just physical shifts. There's an emotional softening, too. Tears have flowed on the mat; laughter has bubbled up after the release of long-held pain. There is power in moving with awareness and intention. I've found that suppleness—through these fascia-based practices—creates space, not just in the joints, but in the mind. It's the feeling of mental clutter dissolving, making room for calm and a renewed capacity to handle stress.

Where to begin? Suppleness starts with hydration and gentle movement. To build suppleness, start by preparing your body's connective tissue with these three practices:

- **Rolling.** Try a tennis ball under your feet or a foam roller for your thighs. Spend two to three minutes per area.
- **Dynamic stretches.** Cat-Cow, arm swings, or ankle circles prep fascia for movement.
- **Hydration hack.** Drink water with electrolytes, such as lemon juice and salt, before rolling to plump tissues.

Then, integrate suppleness into your life by creating short rituals you can do throughout the day, like these:

- **Morning Flow.** Spend five minutes in bed stretching like a cat—reach your arms overhead and point/flex your feet.

- **Desk Reset.** Every hour of the day, try to do seated spinal twists or shoulder rolls.
- **Evening Unwind.** Pair rolling with deep breaths. For example, you can exhale as you release tension.

From Personal Passion to Universal Purpose

As a woman in midlife, I feel more connected than ever to the women and men I serve, many of whom are navigating the same transitions I am. Hormonal changes, joint stiffness, unpredictable energy, and an evolving relationship with the body are all part of the landscape.

My husband and I have made mobility a non-negotiable part of our lifestyle. We often talk about the importance of being resilient for each other, and how this practice is a form of love and an investment in longevity. So, we train, we roll, we walk, we stretch.

That's why, to me, suppleness is more than a pillar of the 4S Method. It's a mission. I want every person who picks up this book to feel empowered to care for their body in a meaningful way. You don't need to be athletic. You don't need to be young. You just need to be *willing*.

Reflection:
Where do you feel stiffness—physical or emotional? How would freedom there change your life?

Chapter 7
SUSTENANCE — FOOD AS CELLULAR MEDICINE

"Every bite of food is a set of instructions—changing your hormones, your brain chemistry, your immune system, and even your genes."
— *Dr. Mark Hyman*

My kitchen became my laboratory long before I ever studied wellness for professional purposes. When doctors couldn't give me answers and my labs kept coming back "normal," I knew something deeper was going on. It was a friend—a naturopath—who first helped me connect the dots. I started to understand the role food plays in my health. And it was either helping me heal or quietly making things worse.

For much of my 20's and early 30's, I stayed current with diet trends, experimenting with many of them in an effort to be thin. I definitely did not understand the role of nutrition. I came to realize what many researchers have known for years: that food is the most powerful daily tool we have to influence how we age, how we feel, and how we function. By changing my priorities from being thin to being nourished at a cellular level, I changed my entire dynamic with food.

And that's what the Sustenance pillar is all about; feeding your body to help your cells thrive! It's embracing anti-inflammatory eating for vibrant aging—by supporting your joints, your energy, your focus, and your mood. Whether you're 35 and feeling new aches or you're 65 and noticing stubborn weight or fatigue, your food choices are influencing everything. The good news? It's never too late to shift course.

The Science of Anti-Inflammatory Eating

As we age, our bodies naturally lose some of their antioxidant power and gain more low-level inflammation—a combo researchers call "inflammaging." This slow, silent inflammation can lead to stiff and achy joints, brain fog, memory slips, and even an increase in belly fat, especially the kind that's hard to lose. (That struggle is real!)

Taking a nutrient-rich approach to eating, such as the Mediterranean diet, which is full of veggies, good fats, and lean proteins, helps counter that. Research has consistently shown that a Mediterranean diet is one of the most powerful ways to calm the body's internal inflammatory "fire." It has been proven to significantly reduce inflammation markers such as CRP33 and is even associated with longer telomeres, the protective caps on our DNA, that are linked to slower cellular aging.[34] In other words, the food on your plate can directly influence how well you age.

Food is more than fuel for the body; it gives it instructions. It literally tells your body what to do. For example, omega-3 fatty acids—from wild salmon or flax, for example—send messages to turn on your "longevity" genes. Olive oil sends messages to your mitochondria—the power plants inside your cells—so they produce energy more efficiently. And prebiotic fibers from foods like garlic, onions, or Jerusalem artichokes feed the beneficial bacteria in your gut, which then create compounds that support immunity and digestion. Every meal is like sending your body a set of instructions—nutrients interact with your cells, your genes, and even your gut bacteria to tell them what to repair, how to produce energy, and how to defend against stress and disease.

Did you know that 70% of your immune system lives in your gut? When your gut lining gets worn down from stress, food intolerances, food allergies, or processed foods, particles can slip through and trigger widespread inflammation, leading to what some refer to as "leaky gut" syndrome.

An anti-inflammatory diet—one that is rich in whole foods, omega-3s, antioxidants, and fiber and that minimizes processed foods, sugar, and trans fats—is generally safe and beneficial for most people. Moreover, people with autoimmune issues often feel better when they remove irritating foods, and research shows that eating a more anti-inflammatory diet can significantly improve digestion, immunity, and energy.

A simple way to accomplish all this while plating your meals is to think of the 50/25/25 plate:

- **50% colorful plants**. Think variety! Aim for 9+ servings of veggies and fruits each day (more veggie heavy)
- **25% clean protein**. Prioritize wild-caught fish, humanely raised poultry, eggs, and beef
- **25% whole grains**. Complex carbohydrates like quinoa, brown rice, or sweet potatoes

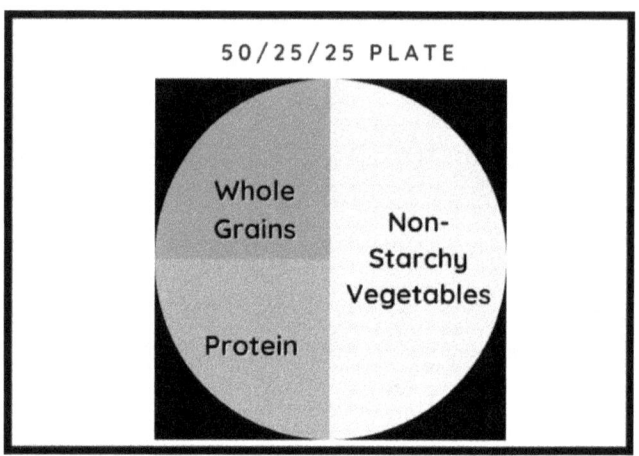

Think of the 50/25/25 plate not as a rigid rule but as your ultimate tool for building a truly anti-inflammatory diet. The template—half non-starchy vegetables (with a little fruit), a quarter lean protein, and a quarter high-fiber carbs—is designed to naturally guide your choices toward foods that fight inflammation—like leafy greens, fatty fish, and whole grains—while minimizing space for the processed foods that can fuel it. By populating your plate with these nutrient-dense foods, you're not just following a ratio; you're actively choosing a powerful, anti-inflammatory way to eat.

This is an evidence-based style of eating, and it is prevention-focused, flexible, and budget-friendly. It has been shown to lower the risk of dementia by more than 50% and to decrease the risk of heart disease significantly. As for flexibility, you don't have to count calories or weigh your food. Just build your plate by proportion. It works with any cultural cuisine—from Mediterranean to Latin to Asian. And when it comes to being easy on your budget, know that frozen berries are just as rich in nutrients as fresh and that canned wild salmon offers powerful omega-3s without breaking the bank.

Where to begin? Try these three small steps:

- **Audit your pantry.** Remove any/all of the boxes and bags of highly processed foods you're storing.

- **Upgrade your breakfast.** Eat a protein-rich breakfast to kick off your day and create lasting energy.

- **Track your wins.** Pay attention to your energy, digestion, and sleep after making changes. Your body will tell you when it's working.

Hydration: The Forgotten Partner

So many of us are carrying around water bottles or jugs of some shape and size these days, as we have learned that hydration is essential. But here's what often gets missed: Not all water is created equal. And water alone isn't enough to hydrate us at the cellular level.

If you're drinking filtered or bottled water without minerals, you might actually be flushing out essential electrolytes rather than replenishing them. Electrolytes, including sodium, potassium, magnesium, and chloride, are vital for nerve function, muscle contraction, energy production, and fluid balance. Even if you're not an athlete, your body still needs them every day, especially if you're under stress, sweating, traveling, drinking caffeine or alcohol, or living in a hot climate.

Prioritize electrolyte-balanced fluids such as coconut water, herbal teas, or water enhanced with trace minerals or natural sea salt. And don't forget hydrating foods like cucumber, watermelon, oranges, and leafy greens; they deliver water and minerals in one refreshing bite.

Hydration isn't just about drinking more; it's about *absorbing* what you drink.

Cellular hydration is fundamental to our health. Here's why:

- Mild dehydration—just 1to 2% fluid loss—has been shown to impair energy production and detoxification.[35]
- 2% dehydration impairs memory and focus.[36]
- Electrolytes (e.g., sodium, potassium, and magnesium) regulate fluid balance.[37]
- Older adults are at higher risk for dehydration because their thirst signals are weaker and kidney function declines, which can lead to dizziness,

fatigue, confusion, and increased chances of heat-related illness or other health complications.[38]

Here's a hydration hack I love to do at the start of each day. Mix a pinch of pink Himalayan salt with a little lemon juice in water. A pinch of salt helps your body hold onto the fluid, while the lemon helps it absorb the water more efficiently, making it especially effective for rehydration.[39]

I also take it to the next level: I make a tray of ice cubes made with filtered water, fresh-squeezed lemon juice, grated fresh ginger and salt. It's so easy to grab and go in the mornings!

The Power of Observing How Food Feels

Sometimes you don't realize how food affects you until you pause and take notice. Instead of battling willpower and strict rules, certain techniques can teach you to observe your cravings without judgment. The simple act of noticing helps break the cycle of impulsive and emotional eating, giving you back a genuine sense of control. It's about working with your mind, not against it.[40]

In fact, learning to be more mindful can fundamentally change your relationship with food. When you become more mindful, you're not restricting yourself—you're reclaiming your own agency.

For years, I dismissed minor symptoms—bloating, fatigue, sinus congestion—as "normal" until I experimented with tracking my meals and reactions. When I started to pay attention, I discovered that dairy foods left me congested for days, that too much sugar usually led to feeling hungover, and that gluten made me bloat and gave me headaches. Making those connections changed everything for me. It was no longer about following a diet; it was about understanding that the foods we eat are in constant conversation with our immune system, our joints, and our energy levels. I was no longer just eating; I was being a diligent observer.

As you begin to pay attention, see if you notice changes like these:

- *Processed foods* and *sugars* might leave you drained, for example, while meals with wild salmon or avocado might feel like they fuel you with steady energy.

- *Gluten* or *dairy* might correlate with sinus pressure or bloating, which are common signs of inflammation.

- *Hydrating foods* like cucumber or oranges might improve your focus even more than stimulants like caffeine.

- *The 50/25/25 plate* has been shown to be anti-inflammatory in studies.[41] You might notice a difference in your body when you eat this way compared to how you feel when you eat more processed foods.

It's important to remember that this isn't about perfection—it's about spotting patterns. If you find that tracking what you eat and how you feel gets stressful, then stop. This should feel like a science experiment, not a test.

Where to begin? Try the following simple approach. For two to four weeks, keep a journal or log of:

- **What you eat.** Include all meals and snacks. For example, you might write "eggs with berries." This is a good opportunity to notice where you choose to eat non-processed foods. For example, choosing eggs for breakfast over a protein bar.
- **How you feel.** You might notice energy spikes or crashes, joint stiffness, sleep quality, mood shifts and other changes. Regardless, write it down.

If you want a structured approach, you might explore elimination diets under professional guidance, but remember, self-observation may often be enough to start.

Client Spotlight

I've participated in Holly's nutrition workshop and left with new tips and methods for healthier eating. Holly is a natural teacher and coach whose holistic approach and expertise provide guidance for total wellness beyond just the movements on the mat.
C.G.

Reflection:
What food leaves you energized? What leaves you drained?

Chapter 8
SERENITY – THE MISSING LINK

*"Almost everything will work again if you unplug it for a few minutes,
including you."*
— *Anne Lamott*

When I first began developing the 4S Method, I knew that movement and strength had to be central to the practice. But something kept whispering to me, something quieter and deeper, that something was still missing. I noticed that so many of my students couldn't seem to be still when they were in savasana—the corpse pose that's often a final resting shape done at the end of practice. They fidget, look at their smart watches or make all sorts of movements when they could be still and allow their whole being to relax and integrate the benefits of what they've just done. I recognized that so many people today can't seem to downregulate their nervous systems; collectively, we have forgotten how to rest and reset. Yet doing so is critical to one's overall health and well-being.

The need for peace and rest became clear to me. From that knowing, the Serenity pillar was born.

The Serenity pillar is about coming home to your body and letting it feel safe enough to rest and repair. In a culture that values productivity over presence and pushing harder over recovery, serenity is both rebellion and restoration. It is the space where resilience takes root.

The Nervous System: The Invisible Foundation

The nervous system is the master communicator of the body. It governs every physiological response from digestion and hormone release to muscle tone, energy, and mood. When our nervous system is dysregulated—that is, chronically stuck in fight, flight, or freeze—everything else suffers. No amount of exercise, supplements, or willpower can override a body in defense mode.

Aging only amplifies this need for regulation. As we age, the nervous system becomes more sensitive, less adaptable, and slower to recover from stress. A review in *Ageing Research Reviews* explains: "Age-related changes in autonomic function can contribute to cardiovascular disease, impaired temperature regulation, and decreased adaptability to stressors."[42] Scientific evidence suggests that with age, the autonomic nervous system declines in function, leading to reduced heart rate variability, a longer recovery time after stress, and a decreased ability to adapt to physiological challenges.[43]

Our ability to handle physical and emotional stress declines with age, thus, aging increases our need to regulate our nervous systems consciously. If we don't, we become even more fragile over time.

However, a growing body of research finds that if we proactively maintain the health of our autonomic nervous system, it will play a key role in healthy aging. Specifically, supporting parasympathetic tone, often called the "rest-and-digest" system, is linked to greater resilience and longevity. As one major review concluded: "Interventions that improve vagal tone, such as mindfulness and slow-paced breathing, have the potential to enhance healthy aging and increase longevity."[44]

This is why serenity is not optional; it is mandatory if we want to move forward in life gracefully, steadily, and with strength and peace.

So, what builds serenity? The following tools do. And they don't require special equipment or hours of free time—just presence.

- **Mindfulness:** This is the practice of paying attention on purpose. Noticing sensations, thoughts, breath. It invites awareness and compassion, which are antidotes to stress.
- **Breath:** Controlled breathing is the fastest, most accessible way to shift your state. As established by neurophysiological research, a slow exhale stimulates the vagus nerve, which activates the parasympathetic ("rest and digest") branch of the nervous system.[45]
- **Stillness:** In a world addicted to doing, stillness is revolutionary. Restorative yoga and yoga nidra offer structured stillness that allows a deep reset.
- **Sound:** Binaural beats at 4–7Hz are theta waves. They have been shown to be an effective, non-pharmacological intervention to reduce anxiety scores by 26% in meta-analyses.[46]

- **Nature:** Time in green spaces improves mood, reduces cortisol, and boosts vagal tone. Forest bathing, even for 20 minutes, has measurable effects on nervous system function and lowering cortisol.[47]
- **Ritual:** Regular practices that ground and soothe, like lighting a candle, drinking some tea in silence, and journaling, train the body to recognize safety.

These tools are more than self-care; they're self-*regulation*. Undeniably, this is something that is terribly lacking in our society today. Almost everyone is wired and tired!

Movement as Emotional Medicine

Not surprisingly, serenity is deeply connected to suppleness. That's because movement—particularly mobility-based movement—is a tool of the nervous system, too.

We hold emotions and stress in our tissues. Our hips, jaw, shoulders, and diaphragm are common storage areas for tension. When we release tension through gentle movement or fascia work, we aren't only "stretching," we're unblocking flow. We're metabolizing our stress and reestablishing a deep-seated feeling of safety in motion.

Mobility builds trust—trust in our bodies and trust in ourselves.

I often tell my students that movement is how the body tells the truth. I can see it in those who can't drop their shoulders from their ears, expand their arms to a "T," or even grasp the back of their leg. One student told me they felt more peace from ten minutes of breath-guided movement than from an hour on their therapist's couch. I'm not criticizing therapy by any means; I'm pointing out the innate intelligence of the body. Mobility, when paired with mindfulness and breath, becomes a very powerful healer for us.

Sleep: The Unsung Healer of Aging

As we age, sleep becomes not just a luxury, but a lifeline. During deep sleep, the brain clears toxins, muscles repair, and vital hormones are released. Yet, aging often disrupts sleep architecture, reducing restorative slow-wave sleep and increasing nighttime wakefulness. Poor sleep accelerates cellular aging, weakens immunity, and heightens inflammation, compounding the very stressors we aim to mitigate through serenity practices. Sleep hygiene becomes important, consisting of cool, dark rooms, consistent rhythms, and mindful wind-downs. It's not just about rest; good sleep hygiene is a direct investment in the resilience of our nervous systems, our cognitive clarity, and our longevity. In the 4S Method, sleep isn't passive; it's where serenity silently works its magic.

Serenity in Practice

I can't write about serenity without sharing how much it matters in my own life. The older I get, the more I notice how quickly my system can spiral if I don't care for it. A poor night's sleep or an overbooked week can knock my nervous system off balance more than it did ten years ago, lupus aside.

Years ago, working to adjust and improve my sleep was my highest priority. I began by treating bedtime not as an afterthought, but as a sacred transition—dimming lights, silencing screens, and honoring the circadian rhythm my body craved. I learned that sleep isn't just downtime; it's when the nervous system repairs, the brain consolidates memories, and inflammation is quieted. Without it, even the most thoughtful serenity practices lose their power.

Serenity had been a missing piece for me for many years, but once I began these practices, they evolved into beautiful, steady habits that continue to ground me, nourish me, and help me feel more connected to myself. It's not an exaggeration to say it's been life-changing for me, affecting how I move and feel in my body and how I show up for myself every single day.

Over time, I've guided clients to build serenity habits for themselves, too, meeting them where they are and showing them how sustainable change begins with small, intentional steps.

That's why I build serenity into every day, not just every week. My rituals aren't long, but they are *sacred*.

My serenity practices

- I start my mornings with some breathwork. I love doing 10 minutes of *nadi shodhana*, alternate nostril breathing.
- Tea without my phone.
- Movement with intention. No music. No distractions.
- Early morning walks with deep listening and no sunglasses.
- Yoga nidra at least three times a week.
- Journaling when things are weighing on my mind.
- Sound baths when I need a reset.

I may not do all of these every day, but I do something. Serenity isn't about being peaceful like a monk all the time; it's about building a relationship with rest, stillness, safety, and your Self.

The more I teach this method, the more convinced I am that serenity is the secret sauce to life! You can be strong, mobile, and well-nourished, but if your nervous system is in overdrive, your body can't fully receive or integrate the benefits. Without a foundation of rest and calm, even the most disciplined wellness routines can feel like more pressure instead of support.

In the meantime, I've witnessed some remarkable changes in my students: transformations that didn't come from a stretch or a rep, but from stillness. I've seen people melt out of chronic tension and pain, not through more effort, but through intentional pausing. I've seen regular students who've consistently resisted savasana finally let go and find rest. I've seen people come home to themselves, sometimes for the first time in years. I feel incredibly privileged to witness these changes.

This pillar, Serenity, holds deep meaning for me because it's what changed *my* life. It reminded me that rest is not laziness; it's intelligence. That softening isn't giving up; it's a conscious act of choosing to stay. It's an act of strength that doesn't shout, but listens.

Serenity is a balm. It is the exhale, the space between the doings. It's the part that whispers to your body: *"You are safe. You are home. You are whole."*

Nervous System First Aid

Serenity is found in pauses, not in achieving some ideal of perfection.

- **Anchor your breath.** Try the "box breath," sometimes called "4-4-4-4" breathing. Inhale for four seconds, hold for four, exhale for four, hold for four. Try it before meals or meetings.
- **Do a sensory reset.** Splash cold water on your wrists, listen to birdsong, or savor a warm cup of tea.
- **Set tech boundaries**. Silence your notifications for 30-minute windows to reduce cortisol spikes.
- **Get Inverted**. Rest with your legs up the wall (Think of your body as making the shape of an "L".) Spending just a few minutes with your feet above your heart can promote a sense of calm.

Your Serenity Toolkit

- **Take a daily pause**. Set a "rest reminder" alarm for one minute of stillness (close eyes, feel your feet).

- **Set up a bedtime ritual.** Dim your bedroom lights 30 minutes before you go to bed. Then use the stress reset flow chart below to fully unwind.
- **Do an emotional check-in.** Journal one sentence: "Today, I found the most ease when…"

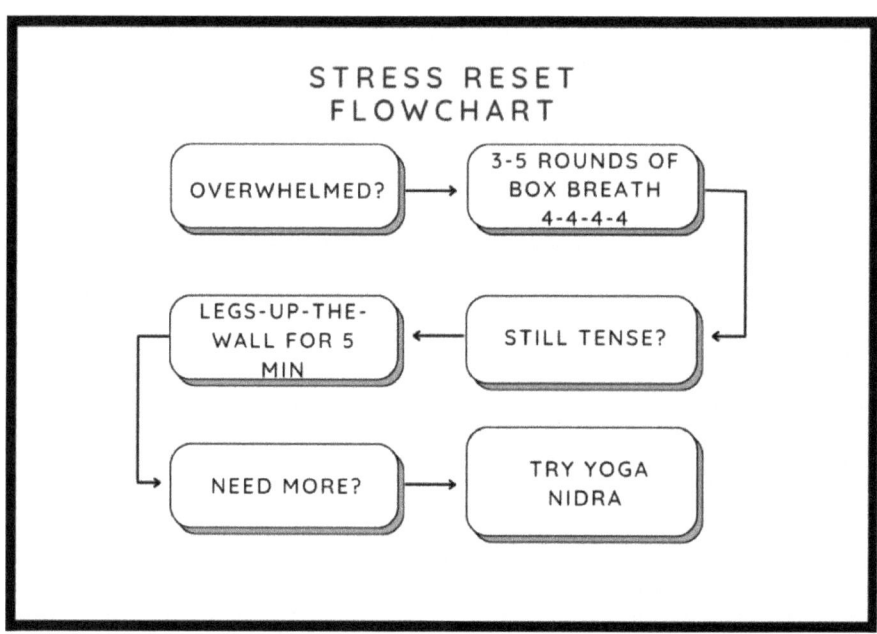

Reflection:
What's your earliest memory of feeling truly at peace? How can you recreate that now?

Chapter 9
POCKET MOVEMENTS

"Better to do something imperfectly than to do nothing perfectly."
— *Robert H. Schuller*

Pocket Movements are my science-backed response to the myth that wellness requires hours and hours of effort. Rooted in research on "exercise snacking" and micro-workouts, Pocket Movements are intentional, bite-sized movements woven into daily life, like desk stretches during work calls or balance exercises while waiting for coffee or brushing teeth. Peer-reviewed studies confirm that even one to five minutes of targeted movement daily can improve metabolic health, build functional strength, and reduce the risk of injury over time. These are the movements that fit into the "pockets" of your time.

For those who want deeper guidance, I've also created the Pocket Movement Library, a growing collection of video tutorials and structured micro-routines organized by the four pillars of the 4S Method. While this book gives you the foundational tools you need, the library serves those who prefer follow-along sessions or want fresh variations each month. Whether you work solely from these pages or explore additional resources, what matters is finding an approach that fits your real life, because consistency with imperfect action always beats perfect plans left undone.

The myth of the perfect wellness routine haunts many of us. In my early fitness days, I felt the heavy weight of guilt anytime I missed a workout. If I had to take a day off or a rest day, I felt like a failure. And I know I'm not alone; so many of us have been conditioned to believe wellness is all-or-nothing and that rest must be earned through exhaustion. And that to progress we must grind on relentlessly.

For years, I operated from a place of *proving* something—to others, to myself, to some vague ideal of what "strong" or "successful" looked like. It took my body's whispers and eventual screams to realize my problem wasn't commitment. It was the myth that fitness had to be hard and "all in" to count.

But I've since learned that balance is a crucial element to support sustainability. And it's something I still consistently work towards. Sometimes I feel grounded; other times, I slip back into old patterns of pushing too hard. Sound familiar? That's why I created Pocket Movements.

The Science of Short-Burst Fitness

We're all short on time. But what if I told you that fitting in just a few minutes of movement actually works? Let's look at the studies that show how valuable those little bursts really are.

• *No more "I don't have time"*
Fact: Around 94% of adults skip workouts because they don't have enough time, but 87% will commit to doing something for less than 15 minutes.[48]
The takeaway: A seven-minute band routine or three-minute desk stretch *is* legitimate. No guilt required.

• *Tiny efforts create big habits*
Fact: A foundational study found that participants who exercised daily for just 5-12 minutes took a median of three weeks to solidify a strong habit, compared to six weeks for those who exercised longer but less frequently.[49]
The takeaway: Frequent, short workouts build exercise habits twice as fast as longer, infrequent ones.

• *Your body loves exercise snacks*
Fact: Twelve-minute sessions three times a week improve insulin sensitivity as much as three times per week.[50] Even one-to-two-minute bursts (like stair climbing) lower heart disease risk by 29%.[51]
The takeaway: Research proves that micro-bursts of movement—as short as one minute—significantly protect your health, making every single effort count. That five-minute hip mobility you do while dinner is cooking? *It counts.*

• *Less guilt, more grace*

Fact: According to a 2019 internal survey by MyFitnessPal, women reported feeling guilty about skipping a long workout more than twice as often as they did about skipping a shorter, micro-workout.[52]

The takeaway: You only did three minutes today? That's three minutes your body didn't get yesterday.

- ***The one-minute miracle***

Fact: Just four and a half minutes a day of vigorous activity, such as stair climbing, reduces mortality risk by 49% in non-exercisers.[53]

The takeaway: Your "I'm too busy" excuse? *Gone.*

Where Pocket Movements Fit in Your Life

Pocket Movements meet you exactly where you are—whether you're:
- managing chronic pain, and you need gentle, adaptive practices
- balancing intense workouts with mobility and recovery
- short on time but crave consistent self-care
- rebuilding strength after an illness or injury, or
- simply wanting a more sustainable approach to movement, active recovery, and rest.

That three-minute seated spinal wave before bed? The wall-supported stretch while your coffee brews? They count. *They all count.* Because showing up for yourself in the pockets of your time compounds— each one is a small investment that builds your physiological resilience, gain by gain, just like the funds in your savings accounts.

Think of Pocket Movements as your wellness allies; they're not there to replace anything. They won't substitute your favorite yoga class or CrossFit session. They'll make them better. That one-minute sigh reset between meetings? It's what keeps you present and grounded. Those five minutes of hip circles at your desk? They're why your Sunday vinyasa feels fluid instead of forced!

The magic of small pockets of time is that they don't demand perfection, and they don't compete with your time, routine, or health challenges. They complement and support them.

4S Method Pocket Movements

Think of Pocket Movements as love notes to your body. Get the details about each of these practices in the Pocket Movements in Action supplement in the back of the book.

- **Strength Pocket Movement.** While your coffee or tea is brewing in the morning, do a five-minute Morning Band Routine.

- **Suppleness Pocket Movement.** Between work calls, do three minutes of a seated cat-cow, moving the spine through flexion (rounding spine back) and extension (rounding spine forward).

- **Sustenance Pocket Movement.** After lunch, take five minutes to do post-meal breathwork, like a few rounds of belly breathing, also known as diaphragmatic breath. To do that, breathe in through the nose for the count of four, exhale through your mouth for a count of six to eight, letting your belly collapse.

- **Serenity Pocket Movement.** Before any stressful task, take one minute to do a Cyclical or Physiological Sigh. Take a long, slow breath in through the nose, filling up about three-quarters of the way. Then take a short, fast breath in through the nose to fill up all the way before exhaling slowly through the mouth. Try to extend the exhale as long as possible.

Pocket Movements aren't about shortcuts; they're about sustainability. They're about giving yourself permission to care for yourself without overhauling your life, permission to trust that small moments compound, and permission to redefine "wellness" as something that fits you now *and* as you age.

Pocket Movements aren't just practical, they're quietly defiant. Every time you choose a two-minute proactive breath reset over a stress-laden reaction, or you prioritize ten minutes of mobility work before pushing through one more tough workout, you're rejecting the myth that wellness requires extremes. This is how we rebel: by caring for our bodies and minds in ways that are well-balanced, sustainable, kind, and unapologetically aligned with real life.

Reflection:
What's one Pocket Movement you can pair with a daily habit, such as doing calf raises while you brush your teeth? Track it for three days and note if and how it changes your energy or mood.

Chapter 10
THE GOOD LIVING CODE

"Aging is not 'lost youth' but a new stage of opportunity and strength."
— Betty Friedan

The Good Living Code is my manifesto for living well *your way.* With the 4S Method as the framework, think of the Good Living Code as a philosophy, and think of Pocket Movements as the everyday practices that bring it to life.

In a culture addicted to hacks, hustle, and extremes, choosing simplicity is the most radical move you can make. This is wellness stripped back to its essence. It's daily practices that cultivate self-trust and offer a return to inward listening. It's leaning into more ease and building consistent time for rest. It's finding joy and freedom in movement. Together, these essentials build vitality from the inside out. Aging well isn't resistance to time; it's rebellion against everything that wastes it.

Here's my truth at the age of 55: I have wrinkles and gray hair. Cellulite. A few post-menopausal or lupus (who knows?) pounds that settled in like uninvited houseguests. And, yes, there are days when fatigue wins. But I also have what the anti-aging industry and the societal norms don't want you to believe is possible: a deep, unshakable friendship with my body. A peace that comes from *balance* rather than *burnout*. And tools to ensure I'll never shrug and say, "I guess this is just part of getting older."

I'm not here to bash other approaches, but to invite you to zoom out and see aging from a more encompassing perspective; to step back to see the bigger picture, and to view aging through a holistic lens. To create a stable foundation built on common sense and science, where practices aren't fads or fixes but sustainable ways of living.

We all have unique stories and challenges, but here's what unites us: the chance to create something more or better without the fear of growing older. Can we examine the structures currently holding up our lives and ask, "Will this truly sustain me for the long haul?" That's the rebellion—choosing the path that allows us to age with strength, grace, and less stress, instead of just surviving the process.

What if 4S becomes your litmus test? Before trying a new longevity supplement or anti-aging hack, before beginning a possibly exhausting workout trend, pause and ask:

- *Will it build **strength** without breaking me?*
- *Will it add **suppleness** to my days?*
- *Will it **sustain** my energy and not drain it?*
- *Will it leave me more **serene**?*

If it won't do *all* of those things for you, it's simply not *good living*. Because good living builds you up and nourishes you, it does not wear you down and deplete you.

This Feels Like a Rebellion

With the 4S Method, we're acting boldly, shunning the norm. Here's how:

We're simplifying in an overcomplicated world. While influencers push ten-step "longevity protocols," we're humming to reset our nerves and rolling our hips with a therapy ball. Research shows people who focused on four or five core habits stuck with them three times longer than those chasing 20+ interventions.[54, 55]

We're choosing presence over performance. No more "no pain, no gain" strategies. Our strength metrics are about carrying groceries without wincing, and our cardio work consists of taking a great hike with a solid elevation gain. (I confess I used to brag about 5:30 a.m. workouts. Now I brag about sleeping until sunrise!)

We're aging loudly. Grey hair? Smile lines? We are confident—and they aren't flaws to fix. Try this: The next time someone says you "look good for your age," smile and say, "I look good *because* of my age."

Every time you opt for a five-minute Pocket Movement—when 45 minutes won't work, or when you respond to your exhaustion without guilt, or when you eat anti-inflammatory foods that fuel you rather than drain you, or when you prioritize sleep over productivity—you're dismantling a system that profits from "grind" culture. This rebellion isn't about perfection. It's about showing up as you are with what you have and holding aging with esteem. After all, it is a privilege some don't get at all.

This is the quiet revolution. No pitchforks needed—just resistance bands, good food, and the courage to trade "never enough" for "more than worthy."

Reflection:
What supposed "wellness rule" do you want to break this week?

THE JOURNEY FORWARD
Good Living is Always Available

As you close this final chapter of the book, take a moment to notice how you feel, not just in your mind, but in your body, your breath, your heart. My deepest hope is that you feel *empowered,* not overwhelmed. That you feel seen, capable, and ready to reclaim your wellness on your terms.

You've learned about the four pillars of the 4S Method—*strength, suppleness, sustenance, and serenity*—not as distant ideals but as living principles you can integrate into your day. Maybe you can start to see movement as nourishment, or find calm in stillness, or simply remember how good it feels to be in your own skin again.

And that's the thing: Good living isn't something you *achieve* once and for all. It's a rhythm. A relationship. A way of being in conversation with your body, your choices, your energy, and your environment.

My advice? Don't overcomplicate it. Start each day with a check-in. A single breath. A moment of stillness. A Pocket Movement. A glass of water. One nourishing action.

Aim for consistency over intensity and awareness over perfection.

And if you fall off track? You start again. That's the beauty of this path; you can always return. Your body is resilient.

Your nervous system is adaptable. Your brain is plastic and ever-changing. You are never stuck unless you decide you are.

Next Steps

While good living is rooted in the 4S Method structure, I invite you to make it your own now. What does *your version* of "good living" look like? Maybe it's taking short walks in nature after lunch. Maybe it's lifting weights with your teenage daughter or your aging father. Maybe it's starting your day without your phone. Or maybe it's journaling before bed or saying No to things that diminish your light.

This is how *wellness* becomes *wisdom.* When the practices you've explored here start to show up in the little details of your daily life—in the way you breathe, the way you stand, the way you respond to stress, the way you recover from challenge.

Let this be your new normal—vibrant, grounded, and self-aware.

Your journey doesn't end here. In fact, this is just one step along a lifelong path of living with more intention, vitality, and ease. The Pocket Movements Library is here as an ongoing resource, a collection of simple, supportive practices you can return to again and again, whether you have five minutes or a full hour. It's designed to meet you where you are, especially on the days when energy feels low. It replaces "all-or-nothing" with balance, especially when time is short.

As you continue, I encourage you to seek out or create your own circle of support, whether it's a local walking group, a yoga class, a friend who shares your wellness values, or even just someone to check in with each week. Community doesn't have to be big or formal to be powerful. When we feel seen, supported, and connected, everything shifts. Wellness becomes more sustainable, and joy becomes more accessible.

And if you ever feel the need for more structure, connection, or guidance, know that I'm here, too. I offer seasonal group programs, one-on-one sessions, and occasional retreats — spaces where you can feel supported, inspired, and part of something bigger. If you are local to Atlanta and want to practice with me, I would love to have you in class at Lift Yoga in Johns Creek. As Helen Keller said, "Alone, we can do so little; together, we can do so much."

Parting Thoughts

Most of all, remember these truths:

You're doing better than you think.
You are capable of so much.
You are allowed to rest.
You are allowed to change.

You are worthy of the wellness you desire.

Thank you for trusting me with your attention, your time, and your intention. I hope this book has been a companion, a mirror, and a gentle nudge toward the life you want to create, not just for a season, but for the long, beautiful, resilient road ahead.

Closing Practice
INTEGRATION MEDITATION

Find a comfortable seat or lie down. Allow your body to rest in a position of ease where you feel supported and stable yet open.

Close your eyes.
Take a full, slow breath in through your nose.
Let the breath go softly out of your mouth.
Allow your breath to anchor you in the here and now.

Now, take a moment to acknowledge the journey you've taken through these pages and through your own inner landscape. You've explored strength, suppleness, sustenance, and serenity. You've listened, stretched, reflected, and *felt*.

Place one hand over your heart, the other on your belly.
With each breath, feel the aliveness of your body.
With each exhale, soften any remaining effort.

Now, in your mind's eye, gently repeat the following:

> *I am strong. I am flexible. I am nourished. I am at peace.*
> *I trust my body. I honor my needs. I walk forward with awareness.*
>
> *Good living is not a destination. It is how I show up, day by day.*

Stay with your breath. Feel the weight of your body on the floor or chair—the gentle pull of gravity, the quiet support beneath you.

When you're ready, invite small movements back—maybe a wiggle through your fingers or toes, or perhaps a soft turn of the head side to side.

Gently open your eyes, returning to the space around you. Know that you carry everything you need within you. You are already on the path.

To support your practice, I've created exclusive companion audio for the meditations in this book. Scan the QR code or visit: https://goodliving-wellness.com/my-book

Supplement
POCKET MOVEMENTS IN ACTION

A practical guide to weaving the 4S Method into your daily life

Now that you know the four pillars of the 4S Method—*strength, suppleness, sustenance,* and *serenity*—it's time to put them into action. In this section, you'll find simple, easy-to-use Pocket Movements that help you move with more ease, restore balance, and support your body every day. Think of these as small, powerful tools that make the 4S Method a part of your life, one movement at a time.

STRENGTH
Five-Minute Morning Band Routine

This combination activates your glutes and shoulders to prevent compensatory movements in your daily tasks. Great to do when the coffee or tea is brewing.

Banded Glute Bridges — 2 minutes

These target your glute medius to protect your knees when you're climbing stairs and lifting things.[56]

1. Loop a resistance band above your knees and lie on your back with your feet hip-width apart.
2. Lift your hips while pressing your knees outward against the band. Squeeze your glutes at the top.

Banded Rows — 2 minutes

These counteract that "computer hunch" and help improve posture.[57]

1. Anchor a non-looped resistance band across your front at waist level and hold the ends with both hands.
2. Pull straight back by squeezing your shoulder blades together, keeping your arms straight. Imagine trying to squeeze a pencil between your shoulder blades.
3. Slowly return your arms to the starting position.

Calf Raises — 1 minute
1. Slowly rise onto your toes and then lower with control.
2. Bonus: Do these when you're brushing your teeth!

SUPPLENESS
Three-Minute Spinal Waves

This combination combats stiffness from sitting and hydrates the spinal fascia. Great to do between work calls or while sitting in a carpool line.

Seated Cat-Cow — 1 minute
- Arch and round your spine rhythmically, emphasizing the full breath.

Side-Bend Twists — 1 minute
- Sit tall and reach your right arm overhead to the left. Twist gently. Then switch sides.

Seated Forward Fold — 1 minute

Hinge at your hips, letting your spine drape. Hold for 30 seconds or more to improve hamstring flexibility and promote muscle relaxation[58]

SUSTENANCE
Post-Meal Breathwork

This breathing technique uses slow, deep breaths to activate the relaxation (parasympathetic) response. For people who experience stress-related bloating or fullness after eating, practicing this consistently can help reduce these uncomfortable digestive symptoms.[59] It works great after any meal.

Diaphragmatic Breathing (Belly Breathing)
1. **Sit** in a comfortable position.
2. **Place one hand** on your stomach and the other on your chest.
3. **Breathe in slowly** through your nose. Feel your stomach push out against your hand. Try to keep your hand on your chest still.
4. **Breathe out slowly** through your mouth with pursed lips—like blowing out a candle. Feel your stomach fall.
5. **Repeat** this for several minutes.

SERENITY
One-Minute Sigh Reset

This is great to do before handling stressful tasks. It rapidly lowers cortisol and resets the nervous system.[60] For an enhanced effect, close your eyes.

Cyclic Sighing — 3-5 rounds
1. **Inhale:** Breathe in slowly and deeply through your nose until your lungs are mostly full.
2. **Second Sniff:** Take a second, shorter inhale through your nose to fully top off your lungs.
3. **Exhale:** Exhale very slowly and audibly through your mouth with a long, sighing sound. Focus on making the exhale as long and complete as possible.

4   **Repeat:** This cycle (double inhale + long exhale) is one round. Repeat for 3 to 5 rounds. This takes about one minute.

Tips for Success

Try these to get even more benefit:

o   **Pair with your habits.** Attach these Pocket Movements to your existing routines. For example, do breathwork after finishing a meal.
o   **Track your progress:** Note any changes to your energy or pain levels in a journal.
o   **Adapt:** Swap the band work for bodyweight if needed.

Scan the QR code below to download your free, 4S Method tracker. Start small, stay consistent, and rebel against "all-or-nothing" wellness!

GLOSSARY

LEGEND

💪	Builds Strength
🤸	Encourages Suppleness
✊	Feeds Sustenance
🖐	Nourishes Serenity
😫	Depletes Strength
🧊	Suppleness at risk, stiff, inflexible
🖐	Sustenance poor
😵	Serenity compromising

A

Anti-inflammatory nutrition (✊ Sustenance)
Nutrition obtained by eating foods that reduce chronic inflammation, including berries, leafy greens, fatty fish (e.g., salmon), and spices (e.g., turmeric). Helps the body heal and age better.

Autoimmunity (😫 🧊 🖐 😵)
A term for when the immune system attacks healthy cells by mistake (e.g., rheumatoid arthritis, Hashimoto's thyroiditis, Multiple Sclerosis, Lupus, Type 1 Diabetes). Managed by:
- **Gentle strength training** (to avoid overstressing the body)
- **Gut-friendly foods** (like bone broth, probiotics)
- **Mobility work** (to prevent stiffness)
- **Stress reduction** (breathwork, meditation)

B

Breathwork (🕊 Serenity)
Deliberate breathing techniques (e.g., inhale 4 seconds, hold 7 seconds, exhale 8 seconds) to lower stress and boost energy.

C

Compound Movements (💪 Strength)
Exercises that use multiple joints/muscles at once (e.g., squats, deadlifts). Great for full-body strength.

Cortisol (😰 🛡 😲)
A stress hormone that harms all Pillars, cortisol is the body's main stress hormone. Chronically elevated levels can:
- Shrink muscles
- Weaken immunity (more colds/infections)
- Make joints stiff and painful

D

Dynamic Mobility (🤸 Suppleness)
Moving joints through their full range *actively* (e.g., leg swings, arm circles). Better than static stretching before workouts.

E

Eccentric Strength (💪 Strength)
Strengthening muscles by lengthening them under tension (e.g., slow 3-second descent in a push-up). Prevents injuries.

Electrolytes (🫴 Sustenance)
Minerals, including sodium, potassium, and magnesium, that are lost when we sweat or when we drink too much water. Needed for muscle cramps, energy, and hydration.

F

Fascia (💪 Suppleness)
The body's "spiderweb" of fibrous tissue that wraps muscles and organs. Gets sticky with stress and dehydration. Needs massage and movement.

Functional Strength (💪 Strength)
Strength for daily tasks (e.g., lifting kids, climbing stairs). Focuses on useful movement patterns.

H

Hormesis (💪 Strength, Suppleness)
Small, intentional stresses, like cold showers or short sprints, that train the body to handle challenges better.

Hydration (🫴 Sustenance)
Not just water—We need minerals like those in coconut water or lemon-plus-salt to absorb water properly and lubricate joints.

I

Inflammaging (🍟 😵)
Chronic low-level inflammation that speeds up aging. Diet and stress control help reduce it.

Leaky Gut (🖐)
When the gut lining gets damaged enough from stress and junk food, for example, it allows toxins into the blood. Repaired with the help of healing foods (bone broth, probiotics).

M

Microbiome (🍚 Sustenance)
This is the name for the trillions of bacteria in your gut that affect immunity, mood, and digestion. Fed by fiber (veggies) and fermented foods (yogurt, sauerkraut).

Mobility vs. Flexibility (💪 Suppleness)
- **Mobility:** How well you *actively control* joint movement (e.g., deep squat).
- **Flexibility:** How far you can *passively stretch* (e.g., touching toes).

Myofascial Release (💪 Suppleness)
Rolling on a foam roller or ball to break up tight spots in muscles/fascia.

N

Non-Sleep Deep Rest (NSDR) (🕊 Serenity)
A short, 10 to 20-minute guided relaxation (like Yoga Nidra) that mimics sleep's restorative benefits.

P

Parasympathetic Nervous System (🕊 Serenity)
The body's recovery state, characterized by a slowed heart

rate and priority given to digestion. Activated by deep breathing, meditation, or calm environments.

Pocket Movements (💪🤸🥗🧘 ~ All Four Pillars!)
Super short (1 to 5 minutes) workouts or stretches you can do anywhere (e.g., wall push-ups, desk stretches).

Progressive Overload (💪 Strength)
Gradually adding weight and/or reps to keep challenging muscles. This is key for growth.

S

Sarcopenia (😩)
The natural decline in muscle mass after 30. Lifting weights is the best prevention.

Serenity (🧘)
Serenity is the intentional practice of managing stress to restore your body and mind. It is "the art of nervous system regulation." Practices that calm the mind and body include breathwork, yoga nidra, and sleep hygiene. In the 4S Method, serenity is the "secret sauce" that lets strength, suppleness, and sustenance work synergistically.

Strength (💪)
Being strong and preserving muscle mass is your body's natural support system for adventure, play, and everyday ease, giving you sustainable power for real life. The 4S approach to strength prioritizes functional resilience over aesthetics—building the capacity to lift grandchildren, open jars, and move through daily life with ease. Focuses on

mindful resistance (bands, bodyweight, or weights) to combat age-related muscle loss and protect joints.

Suppleness (🐢)

This is an embodied state of having fluid, effortless, and readily available control over your movement. It is attained through building mobile joints and hydrated fascia with dynamic stretches, myofascial release, and mindful movement. Suppleness provides fluidity for lifelong movement. Unlike static flexibility, suppleness emphasizes *usable range of motion*—helping you bend, twist, and rise from the floor with grace.

Sustenance (🍱)

Sustenance is the practice of fueling and hydrating your body with intention. It's about giving your body the quality nourishment it needs to rebuild, recover, and thrive from within. Sustenance is enabled by eating and drinking foods that reduce inflammation, support gut health, and optimize energy. It emphasizes anti-inflammatory eating (like the Mediterranean diet) over highly processed foods, proper hydration, and listening to your body's signals—not restrictive rules.

Sympathetic Nervous System (😵‍💫)

The stress response (fast heartbeat, tense muscles). Chronic activation harms health.

Systems Thinking (💪 🧠 🍔 ~ All four Pillars!)
This is the understanding that your body is an interconnected network, not a collection of separate parts, and that every input has a ripple effect that influences every other aspect of your wellbeing. For example, poor sleep can lead to cravings for junk food, which can generate inflammation in the gut.

T
Telomeres (💪 🧠 🍔 🕊️ ~ All four Pillars!)
Protective caps on DNA that shorten with aging. Lengthening them is a key to longevity. They can be lengthened by:

- Antioxidants (berries, dark chocolate)
- Meditation
- Regular exercise

Theta Waves (🕊️ Serenity)
Brainwave frequencies that occur during meditation, daydreaming, or light sleep. Linked to creativity and calm.

V
Vagus Nerve (🕊️ Serenity)
The longest nerve in the body, it connects the brain to the gut. Calms inflammation when stimulated by humming, cold exposure, deep breathing, and more.

Y

Yoga Nidra (🕊 Serenity)

A lying-down guided meditation that resets the nervous system in 10 to 20 minutes. Sometimes referred to as NonSleep Deep Rest.

NOTES

[1] Foster, E. R., Chasen, M., Krok-Schoen, J. L., & Rosko, A. E. (2023). Multimodal interventions for the management of frailty and cognitive function in older women: A systematic review and meta-analysis. *Maturitas*, *167*, 60–69. https://doi.org/10.1016/j.maturitas.2022.10.003

[2] Mosconi, L. (2020). The XX brain: The groundbreaking science empowering women to maximize cognitive health and prevent Alzheimer's disease. Avery, an imprint of Penguin Random House.

[3] Mosconi, L. (2018). Brain food: The surprising science of eating for cognitive power. Avery, an imprint of Penguin Random House.

[4] Mark D. Peterson, Bryan C. Rheaume, and Paul M. Sen, "Resistance Exercise for the Aging Adult: Clinical Implications and Prescription Guidelines," *Medicine & Science in Sports & Exercise*, 2010, https://doi.org/10.1249/MSS.0b013e3181c8543f.

[5] Laura Bridges and Manoj Sharma, "The Effects of Yoga on Balance, Strength, and Mobility in Older Adults: A Systematic Review and Meta-Analysis," *Journal of Aging and Physical Activity* 31, no. 4 (2023): 456–68

[6] Cramer, H., Ostermann, T., Dobos, G., & Lauche, R. (2018). Injuries and other adverse events associated with yoga practice: A systematic review of epidemiological studies. Journal of Bodywork and Movement Therapies, 22(2), 390–399. https://doi.org/10.1016/j.jbmt.2017.04.002

[7] Telles, S., Sharma, S. K., & Balkrishna, A. (2022). Biomechanical analysis of selected yoga postures: Implications for safe practice. International Journal of Yoga, 15(1), 3–12. https://doi.org/10.4103/ijoy.IJOY_114_21

[8] Sherrington, C., Michaleff, Z. A., Fairhall, N., Paul, S. S., Tiedemann, A., Whitney, J., ... & Lord, S. R. (2017). Exercise to prevent falls in older adults: An updated systematic review and meta-analysis. British Journal of Sports Medicine, 51(24), 1750–1758.https://doi.org/10/1136/bjsports-2016-096547

[9] Telles, Sharma, and Balkrishna, Biomechanical Analysis of Selected Yoga Postures.

[10] Jeong, U. C., Sim, J. H., Kim, C. Y., Hwang-Bo, G., Nam, C. W., & Kim, J. (2015). Effects of gluteus medius strengthening on gait, function, and pain in patients with chronic low back pain: A randomized controlled trial. Journal of Physical Therapy Science, 27(12), 3813–3816. https://doi.org/10.1589/jpts.27.3813

[11] Sherrington et al., *Exercise for Preventing Falls*.

[12] Wolfe, R. R. (2006). The underappreciated role of muscle in health and disease. American Journal of Clinical Nutrition, 84(3), 475–482. https://doi.org/10.1093/ajcn/84.3.475

[13] Wang, Z., et al. (2010). Muscle mass, metabolism, and aging: What we know and what we need to learn. *Journal of Applied Physiology,* 110(6), 555–560. https:/doi.org/10.1152/japplphysiol.00549.2010

[14] Akuthota, V., & Nadler, S. F. (2004). Core strengthening. *Archives of Physical Medicine and Rehabilitation*, 85(3 Suppl 1), S86–S92. https://doi.org/10.1053/j.apmr.2003.12.005

[15] Wilke, J., et al. (2018). Is There an Association Between Aging, Fascia, and Flexibility? A Systematic Review. *Frontiers in Physiology*, 9, 1248.

[16] Brosseau, L., et al. (2023). The Ottawa Panel guidelines for managing osteoarthritis with exercise. *Journal of Rheumatology*, 50(2), 172–180.

[17] Kelley, G. A., et al. (2015). Exercise reduces depressive symptoms in adults with arthritis: A systematic review with meta-analysis of randomized controlled trials. *Arthritis Research & Therapy,* 17(1), 121.https://doi.org/10.1186/s13075-015-0643-0

[18] Cooper, R., et al. (2017). Objective measures of physical capability and subsequent health: A systematic review. *Journal of the American Geriatrics Society*, 65(5), 995–1001. https://doi.org/10.111/jgs.14805

[19] Sipilä, S., et al. (2021). Muscle performance in midlife women: The role of menopause and physical activity. *Journal of Cachexia, Sarcopenia and Muscle, 12*(3), 586-597. https://doi.org/10.1002/jcsm.12698

[20] Peterson, M.D., et al. (2010). Resistance exercise for the aging adult: Clinical implications and prescription guidelines. *American Journal of Medicine, 123*(12), 1086-1092. https://doi.org/10.1016/j.amjmed.2010.05.022

[21] Borde, R., Hortobágyi, T., & Granacher, U. (2015). Dose-response relationships of resistance training in healthy old adults: A systematic review and meta-analysis. Sports Medicine, 45(12), 1693-1720. https://doi.org/10.1007/s40279-015-0385-9

[22] Watson, S.L., Weeks, B.K., Weis, L.J., et al. (2018). High-intensity resistance and impact training improves bone mineral density and physical function in postmenopausal women with osteopenia and osteoporosis: The LIFTMOR randomized controlled trial. Journal of Bone and Mineral Research, 33(2), 211-220. https://doi.org/10.1002/jbmr.3284

[23] Cruz-Jentoft, A. J., et al. (2019). Sarcopenia: Revised European consensus on definition and diagnosis. *Age and Ageing*, 48(1), 16–31. https://doi.org/10.1093/ageing/afy169

[24] Riggs, B. L., et al. (2008). A population-based assessment of rates of bone loss at multiple skeletal sites: Evidence for substantial trabecular bone loss in young adult women and men. *Journal of Bone and Mineral Research, 23*(2), 205–214. https://doi.org/10.1359/jbmr.071020

[25] Pontzer, H., et al. (2021). Daily energy expenditure through the human life course. Science, 373(6556), 808–812. https://doi.org/10.1126/science.abe5017

[26] Watson, S. L., Weeks, B. K., Weis, L. J., Harding, A. T., Horan, S. A., & Beck, B. R. (2018). High-intensity resistance and impact training improves bone mineral density and physical function in postmenopausal women with osteopenia and osteoporosis: The LIFTMOR randomized controlled trial. Journal of Bone and Mineral Research, 33(2), 211-220. https://doi.org/10.1002/jbmr.3284

[27] Sherrington et al., *Exercise for Preventing Falls*.

[28] Francois, M. E., et al. (2015). 'Exercise snacks' before meals: A novel strategy to improve glycaemic control in individuals with insulin resistance. Diabetologia, 57(7), 1437-1445. https://doi.org/10.1007/s00125-015-3574-z

[29] Fiatarone, M. A., et al. (1990). High-intensity strength training in nonagenarians. *JAMA, 263*(22), 3029-3034. https://doi.org/10.1001/jama.1990.03440220053029

[30] Ng, T. P., et al. (2015). Nutritional, physical, cognitive, and combination interventions and frailty reversal among older adults: A randomized controlled trial. *American Journal of Medicine, 128*(11), 1225-1236. https://doi.org/10.1016/j.amjmed.2015.06.017

[31] Ng et al., *Nutritional, Physical, Cognitive, and Combination Interventions*.

[32] Wilke, J., Schleip, R., Yucesoy, C. A., & Banzer, W. (2019). Fascia thickness, aging and flexibility: is there an association? *Journal of Anatomy, 234*(1), 43–49. https://doi.org/10.1111/joa.12902

[33] Schwingshackl, L., Hoffmann, G., & Missbach, B. (2017). "An umbrella review of meta-analyses of randomized controlled trials and observational studies on Mediterranean diet and health." *Critical Reviews in Food Science and Nutrition,* 57(15), 3350–3361. https://doi.org/10.1080/1048398.2015.1107022

[34] Crous-Bou, M., Fung, T. T., Prescott, J., Julin, B., Du, M., Sun, Q., ... & De Vivo, I. (2014). "Mediterranean diet and telomere length in Nurses' Health Study: population based cohort study." *BMJ*, 349, g6674. https://doi.org/10.1136/bmj.g6674

[35] Maughan, R. J., & Shirreffs, S. M. (2010). Dehydration and rehydration in competitive sport. *Scandinavian Journal of Medicine & Science in Sports, 20*(Suppl 3), 40–47. https://doi.org/10.1111/j.1600-0838.2010.01207.x

[36] Ganio, M. S., Armstrong, L. E., Casa, D. J., McDermott, B. P., Lee, E. C., Yamamoto, L. M., & Marzano, S. (2011). Mild dehydration impairs cognitive performance and mood of men. *British Journal of Nutrition, 106*(10), 1535–1543. https://doi.org/10.1017/S0007114511002005

[37] Palmer, B. F., & Clegg, D. J. (2016). Electrolyte and acid–base disturbances in patients with diabetes mellitus. *New England Journal of Medicine, 375*(5), 448–459. https://doi.org/10.1056/NEJMra1503102

[38] Kenney, W. L., & Chiu, P. (2001). Influence of age on thirst and fluid intake. *Medicine & Science in Sports & Exercise, 33*(9), 1524–1532. https://doi.org/10.1097/00005768-200109000-00016

[39] Maughan, R. J., & Shirreffs, S. M. (2008). Development of individual hydration strategies for athletes. *International Journal of Sport Nutrition and Exercise Metabolism,* *18*(5), 457–472. https://doi.org/10.1123/ijsnem.18.5.457

[40] O'Reilly, G. A., Cook, L., Spruijt-Metz, D., & Black, D. S. (2014). Mindfulness-based interventions for obesity-related eating behaviours: a literature review. *Obesity Reviews,* *15*(6), 453–461. https://doi.org/10.1111/obr.12156

[41] Estruch, R., Ros, E., Salas-Salvadó, J., Covas, M. I., Corella, D., Arós, F., ... & Martínez-González, M. A. (2013). Primary prevention of cardiovascular disease with a Mediterranean diet. New England Journal of Medicine, *368*(14), 1279–1290. https://doi.org/10.1056/NEJMoa1200303

[42] Roy, S. (2020). Impact of exercise on the autonomic nervous system in the elderly. Ageing Research Reviews, *62*, 101126. https://doi.org/10.1016/j.arr.2020.101126

[43] Monahan, K. D. (2007). Effect of aging on baroreflex function in humans. *American Journal of Physiology-Regulatory, Integrative and Comparative Physiology,* *293*(1), R3–R12. https://doi.org/10.1152/ajpregu.00031.2007

[44] Zulfiqar, U., Jurivich, D. A., Gao, W., & Singer, D. H. (2010). Relation of high heart rate variability to healthy longevity. *The American Journal of Cardiology,* *105*(8), 1181–1185. https://doi.org/10.1016/j.amjcard.2009.12.022

[45] Gerritsen, R. J. S., & Band, G. P. H. (2018). Breath of Life: The Respiratory Vagal Stimulation Model of Contemplative Activity. *Frontiers in Human Neuroscience,* *12*, 397. https://doi.org/10.3389/fnhum.2018.00397

[46] Garcia-Argibay, M., Santed, M. A., & Reales, J. M. (2019). Efficacy of binaural auditory beats in cognition, anxiety, and pain perception: a meta-analysis. Psychological Research, *83*(2), 357–372. https://doi.org/10.1007/s00426-018-1066-8

[47] Hunter, M. R., Gillespie, B. W., & Chen, S. Y. P. (2019). Urban Nature Experiences Reduce Stress in the Context of Daily Life Based on Salivary Biomarkers. *Frontiers in Psychology,* *10*, 722. https://doi.org/10.3389/fpsyg.2019.00722

[48] American College of Sports Medicine (ACSM) & Fitbit. (2018). *ACSM's Health & Fitness Journal,* *22*(5), 5–8

[49] Phillips, L. A., & Gardner, B. (2016). Habitual exercise instigation (vs. execution) predicts healthy adults' exercise frequency. *Health Psychology*, *35*(1), 69–77. https://doi.org/10.1037/hea0000249

[50] Malin, S. K., Nightingale, J., Vella, C. A., Levine, J. A., & Chipkin, S. R. (2023). Twelve weeks of sprint interval training improves indices of cardiometabolic health similar to traditional endurance training despite a five-fold lower exercise volume. *American Journal of Physiology-Endocrinology and Metabolism*, *325*(4), E375-E384. https://doi.org/10.1152/ajpendo.00192.2023

[51] Ahmadi, M. N., Clare, P. J., Katzmarzyk, P. T., del Pozo Cruz, B., Lee, I., & Stamatakis, E. (2022). Vigorous physical activity, incident heart disease, and cancer: how little is enough?. *European Heart Journal*, *43*(46), 4801-4814. https://doi.org/10.1093/eurheartj/ehac572

[52] MyFitnessPal. (2020). *Micro-Workouts Macro Impact: USA Report* [Internal Market Research Survey]. MyFitnessPal, Inc.

[53] Hamer, M. (2022). Association of wearable device-measured vigorous intermittent lifestyle physical activity with mortality. *Nature Medicine*, *28*(12), 2521–2529. https://doi.org/10.1038/s41591-022-02100-x

[54] Fogg, B. J. (2020). Tiny habits: The small changes that change everything. Houghton Mifflin Harcourt.

[55] Baumeister, R. F., & Tierney, J. (2011). *Willpower: Rediscovering the greatest human strength*. Penguin Press

[56] Kang, S. Y., Jeon, H. S., Kwon, O. Y., Cynn, H. S., & Choi, B. R. (2014). Isometric hip abduction using a Thera-Band alters gluteus maximus muscle activity and the anterior pelvic tilt angle during bridging exercise. *Journal of Electromyography and Kinesiology, 24*(3), 318–324. https://doi.org/10.1016/j.jelekin.2014.01.008

[57] Choi, J.-H., Kim, N.-J., & Kim, D.-Y. (2015). The effects of scapular stabilization-based exercise therapy on pain, posture, flexibility and shoulder range of motion in chronic shoulder pain patients. *Journal of Physical Therapy Science, 27*(12), 3659–3661. https://doi.org/10.1589/jpts.27.3659

[58] ACSM. (2018). ACSM's Guidelines for Exercise Testing and Prescription (10th ed.). Philadelphia: Wolters Kluwer

[59] Ghoshal, U. C., Verma, A., & Misra, A. (2020). Effect of diaphragmatic breathing on symptoms of functional dyspepsia: A randomized controlled trial. *Indian Journal of Gastroenterology, 39*(2), 171–178. https://doi.org/10.1007/s12664-020-01023-0

[60] Balban, M. Y., Neri, E., Kogon, M. M., Weed, L., Nouriani, B., Jo, B., Holl, G., Zeitzer, J. M., Spiegel, D., & Huberman, A. (2023). Brief

structured respiration practices enhance mood and reduce physiological arousal. Cell Reports Medicine, 4(1), 100895. https://doi.org/10.1016/j.xcrm.2022.100895

Acknowledgments

This book began as a personal journey but has only come to life because of the incredible community that has surrounded me with guidance, encouragement, and love. The 4S Method reflects my own lived experiences, yet every chapter carries the influence of those who believed in me, challenged me, and walked alongside me. To each of you, I offer my immeasurable gratitude.

To Steven, my best friend, partner, and the most supportive husband one could ask for, "*Thank you*" does not come close to expressing my gratitude. You have stood by me steadfastly through every endeavor over the last 30 years, embracing with unwavering support my many flaws, my constant "cooking something up" (whether food in the kitchen, creative projects, endless hours on the computer or the sheer busy-ness that I always seem to get myself into), and my deepest desire for us to live as healthfully as possible for as long as possible.

To our four beautiful children, Shawn, Melissa, Michael, and Matthew: I hope you know that I am proud of each of you—not for any specific words or actions, but for creating lives you want to live fully. My greatest hope is that I can make you proud by showing up in my own life with authenticity and purpose, and that, in some way, I can offer an example worth following. I love you all so fiercely!

I am endlessly grateful to Sage Rountree, whose wisdom and mentorship have shaped me as both a teacher and a human. Long before I became a yoga teacher, I was reading her books, inspired not only by her knowledge but by her ability to make yoga feel both practical and accessible. Over the years, I had the privilege of working with Sage as she brought her trainings to the studio I called home. She has become a true role model for aspiring teachers, and our shared Buffalo roots—and wicked sense of humor—only deepen my sense of kinship with her. Having her words open this book is more than an honor; it feels like a full-circle moment in my journey.

This book is undoubtedly stronger thanks to the thoughtful contributions of those who helped shape it. My deepest thanks to Diane Eaton for her patient and insightful editing, and for encouraging me to both trust and expand my voice. I'm deeply grateful for your time and diligence.

I first experienced Sheila Ewers' transformative teaching in 2020 under a large outdoor tent. Her guidance didn't just move my body; it touched my heart. I didn't know then that I would have the fortune not only to work with her but to call her my friend. Early on, she said, "Oh, I would just love to work with you," a statement I initially misunderstood. She wanted more for me than I wanted for myself; she was challenging me to find my voice and value myself before giving all my time and energy to others. Her no-nonsense, tell-it-like-it-is guidance is something I came to deeply respect and appreciate. Without her support and encouragement, this book would not exist.

Major thanks and eternal hugs to Sonya Kuropatwa, the artistic genius behind this book's cover design. You somehow pulled the ideas from my brain, made it a thousand times better, and brought it to life. Thank you for your talent, your time, and for our countless "back and forth" emails and texts. I'm not only grateful for your artistry on this project, but for the creative partnership and friendship we've built co-leading Lift's 200-hour yoga teacher training. This collaboration, like that one, is a joy.

To my students and clients, the heartbeat of the 4S Method: *Thank you*. Every class, session, and conversation has deepened my understanding of resilience and well-being. Hearing that you move and feel better after our time together is a priceless gift and the very reason I love this work. Without you, these ideas would have remained concepts; you brought them to life.

My deepest thanks to Lori Denton, my friend and owner of Lift Yoga. I am grateful for all of the opportunities afforded to me as Director of Operations and as a member of an incredible teaching staff, for the all-out effort (with tears and laughter) we poured into growing Lift over our four years together, and for a friendship that transcends it all.

To my small and mighty circle of friends— *Thank you*. Thank you for the listening ears, the celebrated milestones, and the laughter exactly when needed. For every walk (weighted vest or not), coffee, and delayed dinner date: I'm so grateful for you.

While this book carries my name, it also bears the fingerprints of every teacher, student, colleague, friend, and family member who has walked with me. Thank you for believing in me and for your support when I needed it most. You are the living proof of this book's core belief: that healing and wellness are not destinations to be reached, but a continuous practice cultivated and further enriched in community.

www.ingramcontent.com/pod-product-compliance
Lightning Source LLC
Chambersburg PA
CBHW052033030426
42337CB00027B/4979